Welles-Turner Memorial Library
a department of the Town of Glastonbury
Glastonbury, Connecticut

Cornelia H. Nearing
Memorial Collection

Corneila H. Nearing (1871-1959) was a fine artist and a great citizen of Glastonbury. She loved and used our library and was a great believer in sharing resources. The citizens of Glastonbury continue to enjoy the benefits of her generosity through an endowment she established for the Library. It is from those resources that this book has been purchased for your use and enjoyment.

The Fog
of Paranoia

The Fog of Paranoia

A Sister's Journey through Her Brother's Schizophrenia

SARAH RAE

ROWMAN & LITTLEFIELD PUBLISHERS, INC.
Lanham • Boulder • New York • Toronto • Plymouth, UK

Published by Rowman & Littlefield Publishers, Inc.
A wholly owned subsidiary of The Rowman & Littlefield Publishing Group, Inc.
4501 Forbes Boulevard, Suite 200, Lanham, Maryland 20706
www.rowman.com

10 Thornbury Road, Plymouth PL6 7PP, United Kingdom

British Library Cataloguing in Publication Information Available

Library of Congress Cataloging-in-Publication Data

Rae, Sarah, 1984–
  The fog of paranoia : a sister's journey through her brother's schizophrenia / Sarah Rae.
     pages cm
  Includes bibliographical references.
  ISBN 978-1-4422-2063-8 (cloth : alk. paper) — ISBN 978-1-4422-2064-5 (electronic)
1. Rae, Pat—Mental health. 2. Rae, Sarah, 1984– 3. Schizophrenics—Family relationships—Case studies. 4. Brothers and sisters—Mental health—Case studies. 5. Family psychotherapy—Case studies. I. Title.
  RC514.R27 2013
  616.89'8—dc23
2013016921

Printed in the United States of America

Contents

Introduction

There are over four thousand surveillance cameras on Fourteenth Street alone.[1] When I go outside, day or night, I'm never unobserved. There's always someone over my shoulder. My lead-footed upstairs neighbors stomp around and seem to move furniture at all hours of the night. Sometimes cars, even cabs, pull up under my front window and just sit there for hours until they go back to work. Strangers in New York City can be confrontational, butting in and inviting themselves into your day-to-day activities. These are not things I dwell on, merely facts. But I wonder if some day all of that will mean more to me than it should. If not me, then what about my children? Schizophrenia looms over a family, climbs the family tree and dangles haphazardly, waiting to one day land on someone's back.

When my older brother Pat began having delusions and eventually started accusing us of conspiring against him, I had trouble getting him the help he needed. At first he was only worried about people speaking Spanish around him because he thought they were talking about him. Those delusions slowly built up. Eventually he was convinced people were watching him, going through his things at work, and talking about him behind his back. Sometimes he accused me of letting people into the house when he was at work so they could put cameras and listening devices around his living space. He believed both people he knew and perfect strangers were invading his privacy.

He didn't know why, but he wanted answers. He was beside himself trying to figure out who *they* were and why *they* were after him.

I had trouble convincing others that there was cause for concern because his symptoms would flare up and then slowly dissipate. He might raise concerns about people talking about him behind his back, but then he'd go back to doing his work or going to class as if it didn't bother him anymore. Sometimes he was very agitated and worried about new coworkers, new maintenance personnel, or other changes, but other people in our lives failed to notice.

Even on days when he didn't seem to have a care in the world, his life at home was still very unusual. He would rarely sleep. When he did, he slept on the sofa in the living room because from that vantage he believed he would wake up if anyone tried to come in the door. His hygiene was deteriorating, although he appeared presentable when he would go to work or to the store. I seemed to be the only person who saw that he just wasn't himself any more.

At that time, Pat was seeing a psychiatrist, but Dr. Hollis would not return my phone calls. He diagnosed Pat with attention deficit disorder. Finishing his last semester of college, Pat seemed to be having trouble concentrating on his assignments. I didn't understand; he had never had attention problems before. Hollis gave him a prescription for Adderall (amphetamine and dextroamphetamine) that should have lasted him a month, but he would finish within ten days. It was a popular drug among college students. It helped them stay up late studying or writing term papers and gave them an extra buzz if they drank alcohol with it.

Pat had gotten the drug from friends in order to study for finals when he first started college. He always enjoyed the boost it gave him. So I was sure he had put on a show to convince Hollis to prescribe it for him. I didn't believe that lack of attention was the problem. I assumed he was having trouble studying because the work was getting progressively harder and more advanced, and frankly it's not very fun to write a thesis. Little did I know that impaired attention is a feature of schizophrenia.

Everywhere Pat went he thought people were talking about him, watching him, or even laughing about him. He felt that everyone he saw had intimate knowledge about him and was keeping something from him, something important. He had formerly seen a psychologist named Dr. Milner for social anxiety. Milner was an older man, and Pat always had a great deal of respect for him. He hadn't seen him in at least a year, but knowing how concerned I was, Pat made another appointment with him. I spoke to Dr. Milner after the session, and he assured me that Pat wasn't crazy. He said he was just *acting out* because I was moving to New York City for graduate school. He knew how close we were, and he thought Pat just didn't want me to go. I was speechless. My brother and I were very close, but we talked about things. We didn't hide things from each other and act out for attention. In fact, Pat was usually pretty blunt with me about his feelings. I didn't want to argue with the doctor, but the idea was preposterous. Besides, Pat had never behaved this bizarrely before. He wouldn't even speak outdoors.

Dr. Milner said he had taken Pat to a grocery store where they walked around, and he had assured him that no matter what his instincts were telling him, no one knew him and no one was talking about him or wished him any harm. He said Pat resisted but eventually gave in and agreed with him. I knew this had to be wrong. I had tried many times to talk Pat out of his strange beliefs, but all we did was talk around in circles for hours. When I would ask who would want to spy on him, Pat would answer, "I don't know. Why don't *you* tell *me*?" His feelings were his guide, his proof, and he didn't come home from the appointment feeling any differently.

After a year of Pat's strange behavior, he finally confided in our Uncle Larry that he was convinced someone at work was tapping his phone, sifting through his e-mails, and checking his messages. Larry went to the boss, who also happens to be our dad. Mom and Dad both knew that Pat had been acting differently lately. In fact, one night Dad stood in our kitchen trying to talk Pat out of a delusion. "But why would someone be breaking into the house, Pat? What for?"

"To put bugs and chips in places so they can watch me," Pat replied. "I feel like they put something in my head, transmitting my thoughts. I think everyone can hear my thoughts."

Dad went home that night very scared and weary, but the next day Pat seemed to be on an even keel. He didn't talk about these things all the time. It made it easy for others to turn a blind eye. I guess I didn't have that luxury because we lived together.

When Pat wanted to confront a coworker he believed was watching him and going through his things, Dad asked him to stay home from work a few days. Mom scrambled to contact Dr. Hollis and managed to get a group appointment. Pat, Mom, and Dad sat down to talk with Dr. Hollis about everything that had been going on. He diagnosed Pat with paranoid schizophrenia and gave him a prescription for an antipsychotic called quetiapine, trade name Seroquel.

There are three subtypes of schizophrenia depending on the symptoms of the patient. The paranoid subtype has a preoccupation with delusions or hallucinations, but other symptoms such as disorganized or catatonic behavior, flat or inappropriate affect (i.e., facial expressions), and disorganized speech are not present or at least are not prominent. The disorganized subtype, on the other hand, has prominent disorganized symptoms. This includes erratic behavior, nonsensical thoughts, or disorganized behavior (messy appearance, confrontational behavior).

The disorganized subtype has trouble carrying out many daily activities. In graduate school, my psychopathology professor asked us if we had ever gotten on the subway and witnessed an individual in old, dirty clothing, maybe even with paper shoes or a makeshift hat, carrying a bunch of plastic bags or maybe wheeling a cart of unidentified objects around, some of them found items or simply garbage. The person likely talked to him- or herself, or maybe even sang. What they said was unintelligible, sounded like their own language, or was otherwise incoherent. While those around them noticed their behavior, the individuals seemed unbothered, in their own world. "This," my professor said, "is the disorganized schizophrenic."

The third and last subtype is catatonic schizophrenia, which is characterized by a great deal of movement dysfunction. It is dominated by motor immobility, or its extreme opposite, excessive motor activity. The catatonic schizophrenic can be found stuck in unusual positions. Posturing includes resistance to being moved, irregular or uncomfortable postures, prominent mannerisms, or echopraxia, the repetition of another person's movements. They may display echolalia (i.e., repeating other people) or even mutism. It brings to mind a psychiatric patient, no doubt something I've seen in movies, who shuffles about aimlessly, gets lost in a trance, and cannot accomplish simple everyday tasks.

Given the range of the schizophrenia spectrum, Pat's problems seemed small and relatively promising by comparison. In fact, once we had the diagnosis and medication in hand, it seemed like it would be the end of it all—the end of being woken up in the middle of the night and accused of letting people into the house to spy on him, of spending hours trying to convince him that his suspicions were unfounded, and of rushing out of restaurants and parties to get home and make sure he was okay. But it was just the beginning. It can take a long time to find the right medication and the right dosage. Every case is different.

We learned that the anosognosia associated with the illness leads some patients to go off their medication entirely. Anosognosia means a lack of insight into their disease. Patients may not recognize they have a mental illness or specifically believe they don't have schizophrenia. It's not like bipolar disorder where patients may stop taking medication because they miss the euphoric mood they felt during the manic phase of their illness and are willing to risk the lows that follow. In schizophrenia, patients may not think they need medication at all. They fail to make a connection between their medication and improved health even after years of experience with remissions and relapses into episodes of psychosis.

Not only did Pat not acknowledge his diagnosis, but he didn't believe he needed medication. Because he was not seeing Dr. Milner on a regular basis, no one realized this. He was just given the medication and sent on his way, with no follow-ups to find out how he was responding to the drug. Within a year of his diagnosis, he decided not to refill his medication and quickly relapsed back into active psychosis. It took much longer this time to retrieve him from the fog of his illness.

The prodromal phase of schizophrenia includes the decrease in normal functioning that leads up to the onset of the illness. The active phase includes psychosis and positive symptoms such as hallucinations and delusions. They are called positive symptoms because they feature the addition of abnormal functioning rather than just the loss of normal functioning and they are not present in people who do not have schizophrenia. Cycling out of active psychosis, there is the residual phase highlighted by negative symptoms, such as impaired cognitive function, social withdrawal, apathy, monosyllabic speech, blank expressions, and anhedonia (i.e., the inability to feel pleasure from activities once enjoyed). These are referred to as negative symptoms because they denote a loss or impairment of normal functioning. Remission is the state of having only minimal symptoms. If the state of remission is consistent over time and the patient is able to function well socially, return to work, and assume other everyday living responsibilities, they are considered recovered. Traditionally recovery would mean no more positive symptoms or hospitalizations, but that might not be a realistic way of looking at things, as we will discuss in this book.

Stopping medication is the most common cause of relapse in schizophrenia. Each time a schizophrenic relapses into active psychosis, the possibility they will recover becomes more remote. After Pat's relapse, he became medication resistant. We spent six years trying new medications. As time went by, I witnessed the end of him leaving the house, playing his guitar, and even bathing.

As his old friends reached their thirties and invited me to their weddings, my mom would have flashes of anger, resentment that they had grown up with their minds intact. I reminded her that they had lost a friend and that they would never forget that. When a loved one suffers from schizophrenia, everyone loses something different, whether it was a best friend, a confidant, a sociology tutor, a ray of sunshine, or a dutiful son. Without stories shared by other families like mine, I don't think I could have made it through the grief, the anger, or the confusion to a certain acceptance that, while Pat will never be cured, he will always have me. In 2009, three years after his diagnosis, still looking for answers and peace of mind, I began a master's program in psychology. Insanity might have whisked him away to some far-off unreality where I cannot entirely rescue him, but insanity never met a more devoted sister.

When Pat was diagnosed, I began sifting through my memories looking for a sign. Were there warnings that we missed? Was there some event in his past that changed everything? What could we do to help him now? This book is the result of searching for those answers. It is a culmination of my memories, journal and blog entries, medical records, scholarly articles, and information I was exposed to at NAMI (the National Alliance on Mental Illness). I write under a pseudonym, and other names have been changed to protect privacy.

This is but one family's story, not a blueprint for schizophrenia or the changes that come in its wake. While there is still so much to uncover about this mental illness, my hope is that this book can be a source of comfort and hope.

Part 1

LIFE BEFORE
THE DIAGNOSIS

1

Normal Children

The Raes were a typical middle-class family. My dad's grandfather helped him build a two-story house that we couldn't afford to furnish. We had a big yard with a sandbox, tree house, and tire swing. Dad worked. Mom stayed home until I went to first grade. Before they were thirty years old, they had two children, a boy and a girl. We had a van, a car, a dog, and a cat. We didn't have a lot of money, but I can't remember ever wanting for anything.

I must have heard a million times how different I was from Pat. To this day, I don't buy it. I think people wanted to split us into types; after all, a boy and a girl aren't meant to be the same, particularly in the South. I was slow to warm up. He was easy. I was shy. He was boisterous. There must have been some common ground because we usually got along. Besides the vitiligo on Pat's chest, which went into remission when he was five, we were perfectly healthy kids. We were normal. We started out normal.

Pat was a little over two years old when I was born. I assume he wasn't too excited about having a baby sister. One day, still a newborn, I was sitting in my car seat waiting to go for a ride when our parents caught Pat peeing on me. As we got older, he made small sacrifices to show he didn't despise me. I can't recall him ever taking my "blanky," the security blanket I used for impromptu naps on my toys. He gave me his girl G.I. Joe figurines. He told me jokes. At times he'd let me try to play with his friends without immediately kicking me out of his room.

If we roughhoused and he hurt me, he always looked genuinely sorry. That's something about older brothers. They rail against you and want you out of their way, but they never mean to actually hurt you. I can remember the expression of confusion, of searching for the right thing to say or do to make it better again. He spent just as much time trying not to unsettle me as he did trying to annoy me.

Our house was typically quiet. You'd never know kids lived there. We'd be off playing by ourselves somewhere, sometimes even in a closet for privacy. We were described as "quiet and creative." We threw maybe a handful of tantrums and never in public. In hindsight, we were good as gold. I enjoyed having my toys to myself. I can remember going into a closet to play with Barbie in the afternoon and realizing when I came out again that it was now nighttime.

In the evening, we'd have dinner and then settle into the living room to watch TV. *It's Gary Shandling's Show, Cheers, Dear John,* and *Night Court* were way over my head as a kid, but canned laughter always kept me interested. Pat and I didn't have a bedtime. The four of us cozied up in the living room, enjoying just being together. We kids usually fell asleep around ten o'clock, and Dad would eventually carry us to bed. The idea of staying at another kid's house and putting on pajamas before sundown was very depressing for me. It often seemed like my parents were able to make exceptions for us. Even today they would say we didn't have a bedtime because we were exceptional children who didn't need to be treated that way. Our parents were very in tune with what we could and couldn't handle. They weren't worried about us seeing something on TV that was too mature for us. I could always ask them about things I didn't understand, although they wouldn't always answer me truthfully. Until I was much older, television had me convinced that the act of having sex was simply rolling around naked under the covers with another person.

One thing we had in common was that we were both fickle. We might love a cartoon or a toy tremendously, and then one day we were just over it completely. You could never tell if we'd play with that toy, watch that television show, or eat that cereal again. Well, that's not entirely true. Pat would eat anything. He was always a heavy kid. As an adult he described what it was like: "I just never felt full. For as long as I could remember, I would stop eating only because Dad had stopped eating."

Once one of our grandmother's friends called him "little John Goodman." That hurt his feelings, which in turn hurt mine. I was that kind of little sister. Nobody messed with my brother. To this day the woman's name strikes a nerve in me. That was how close we were as little children. Neither of us liked to see the other put out, unless one of us was the one doing it.

We were competitive. In camp, there was an annual swimming competition called Down the River. Pat beat me every year. He could swim laps long after I gave up, my eyes swollen from the chlorine. He was ranked a "porpoise," and I was a "fish." The following year I swam a little harder and was ranked a "shark." Still I was disappointed I couldn't match my brother's rank. I decided the next year I just wouldn't get out of the pool until he did. And finally I made it to porpoise: forty-eight laps of a twenty-five-yard pool. I was nine years old. There were no other children my age still in the pool when I finished. Pat's reaction was, "So what?" I was always trying to make him proud, and being the little sister of an athletic kid meant really pushing myself.

Kids at camp ranged from age five to twelve. We were split into groups by age and, in Pat's case, size. He was tall for his age, and counselors thought it would be unfair and maybe dangerous for him to play sports all day with kids half his size. Once a week the whole camp, all the groups, came together to compete. Each kid belonged to one of two tribes. The Powhatan and Choctaw tribes would compete in a relay race that included every event that existed at camp: swimming, tennis, riflery, mini-golf, flag football, basketball, and others. The majority of campers didn't participate but rather stood on the sidelines in full tribe regalia and cheered on the competing tribesmen. The revelers started out in the gymnasium while competitors took their positions. Then they spilled out into the yards and pavilions as we proceeded from event to event.

Pat usually played some part in the games, but I was neither athletic nor comfortable in a leadership role. My counselor asked me to represent the Choctaw in pottery. This meant getting the red baton and spinning a perfect bowl faster than my opponent. When the judge gave me the okay, I'd have to cut it from the wheel, put it in the kiln, and then run like hell to the next event to hand off the baton. Coach Cameron, who would later be my swim coach in middle school, was the officiator. The Powhatan kid and I were neck and neck. Then Coach blew the whistle and said, "Rae, you're finished. Move out." I ran out of that ceramics barn, grabbed the baton from another sweaty camper, and struggled to hang onto it with all the wet clay on my hands. I had never been so exhilarated. I heard all the other campers cheering me on, but I only heard Pat's voice telling me to go, go, go. The Choctaw won that year.

I was always competing with Pat. I used his intelligence to gauge how smart I should become within the next two years. I listened to him talking with our father about things like football and music and made a mental note. Sometimes it felt like I'd never catch up, and then I finally got a chance to shine. I was in second grade, crossing the Causeway with my family. The Causeway toll bridge is twenty-four miles across Lake Pontchartrain, and on the way home in the evening we could see the sun setting pink and purple behind the swamps in Manchac.

My dad was joking, telling me that the sun was setting into the lake. "Look, you can see the bubbles! It's boiling!" My brother agreed with him, nodding furiously, but little did they know that I had just learned about the solar system in school. "No it doesn't," I said. "The sun is far, far away." But I still looked closely for bubbles.

Like most older brothers, Pat was usually able to escape trouble for scaring me or telling me off. Mom would usually roll her eyes. Pat would roll his too. It's like they had a secret language of brushing me off. Dad, on the other hand, was always trying to get Pat to care for me more. In Dad's mind he should be protective of his little sister, not "accidentally" hitting her in the head with a tennis racket. "Hug your sister and tell her you're sorry," Dad would say. Pat would wrap an arm around me begrudgingly, wrinkling his nose to show his disgust. It made me sublimely happy.

I'd take social cues from him, if he'd let me, and he took his cues from our parents. It wasn't easy to get praise in our house. It required a great deal of intuitiveness and planning. Being funny and clever were definitely the most desirable qualities. Being a boy also helped.

I vividly remember having holiday parties at our house. I wasn't even in first grade yet. We would all eat together and then the men would retire to the den, sipping cocktails and unbuckling their belts to accommodate full bellies. They'd watch television, tell jokes, laugh loudly, and nap. The women were in the kitchen, but Mom was the one doing all the cleaning up. The women would say mean things about people, maybe about my cousin's new girlfriend or about how much my grandfather ate. It was trash talk, gossip, cattiness. You didn't have to be grown up to wonder, what do they say about me when I'm not around?

I could sense my mom's disappointment. She was just going through the motions, listening to Dad's family, dutifully cleaning their dirty plates. I stood on the threshold between the kitchen and the den. Listening to both rooms, I looked mostly for smiles. It seemed infinitely better in the den than in the kitchen. Pat was there, curled up on a pillow on the floor and laughing with the men. I saw him as my equal and thought that I should get to sit in the den too, even if I was a girl. I should get to pick. But part of me felt like less of a girl, less of a female, if I didn't cluster with the women in the kitchen.

In the den, Pat would goof off and make people laugh. He seemed to me to be part of the gang, fitting in perfectly. Today, I'm sure I would view it much differently if I could go back in time to 1989. Pat was a warm, friendly kid. He was popular and he was fair. It meant that everyone knew him and liked him, but you better not cut in front of him in line at the water fountain. He liked to tell jokes and do impressions. What my extended family was doing, though, was laughing at him, not with him. Over the years, Pat would realize this, and when they asked, "Pat, do that impression I like so much, do Elvis," he would flatly decline. He lost a great deal of innocence once he realized it was ridicule. He became sensitive to the possibility that people were taking advantage of him. His jokes went from impressions to bitter sarcasm. He used to be quite optimistic and happy-go-lucky. Paranoia wasn't built into him.

I clung to my mother the first couple of weeks of preschool. She would hand me off to the teacher, and I would cling to her. After she left, Mom would call to see if I was okay. "She's fine now. She's playing." Still I always dreaded the first day of school each fall. I've always been a classic introvert. Being around too many people makes me tired after a while. Literally, it zaps the energy out of me. The less I know a person, the more exhausting it is. I have to get some time alone. That's one thing my mother and I have in common. We look forward to an evening alone, a morning to ourselves, a quiet space to gather our thoughts. It's like recharging a battery. It takes a long time in solitude before I feel the least bit stir-crazy. But if I spend too much time at home, leaving the house gets *weird*. Other people will make me anxious and fidgety. I read too much into the expressions and demeanor of strangers I pass on the street or in the subway.

Other people, extroverts, derive energy from being around people. Pat was more like that. He made friends easily, he liked being with people, and he met social situations head on. Our attitudes weren't entirely matched by our parents. Dad had the playful sense of humor that Pat had, but he was emotionally sensitive like me. There were two speeds with Dad, pensive and quiet or silly and playful. When he came home from work, it was like a bell went off in our heads. Playtime! He would pick me up, flip me over, and lift me so that my feet would touch the ceiling. Then he would jog around the house that way, letting me "walk" on the ceiling.

Mom was quiet, usually an observer. She was the rock, the one who always had her feet on the ground. There's a home movie where my dad interviewed me at age four. He asked me how old I thought he was, and I said he was eight years old. He asked how old Mom was, and I said she was eleven. He always joked that meant he looked younger than Mom, but it was more about him being like a kid, whereas she was the adult in the house. She rolled her eyes at the three of us a lot.

We did well in school. I was always an advanced student, taking English and math a grade above my peers. Pat grew into his grades, making more As as time went by. His brain loves a challenge. The bigger the challenge, the more involved Pat is and the more attention he gives it. He could break something down to its basic parts so that even someone younger like me or someone without any knowledge in the subject could understand it. He still tries to do this sometimes, but his mind isn't so reliable anymore. Some of his negative symptoms (called negative because they refer to a deficit in cognitive functioning) include difficulty sustaining attention and poor "executive functioning"—that is, the ability to absorb and interpret information and make decisions based on that information. Add to this the fact that he is cut off from the world, from the news and the buzz, when he is withdrawn in the residual phase of his illness. He takes no interest in it. In March 2011, he asked me if Obama had passed health-care reform, which had passed the year before.

We went to an excellent school. It was private and stressed discipline and intellect above all else. It seemed easy to learn when surrounded by ardent learners, other kids with a healthy appetite for knowledge.

I remember my grandfather, Grandpa Howard, mentioning how high we had scored on standardized tests. I can't be sure, but I think our school used the Otis-Lennon School Ability Test. Funny thing is, no one had told us we did well. What Grandpa said was news to us. The scores and how to read them had been mailed to our parents, who in turn proudly showed them to other people. But they never said anything to us about it. Without meaning to, because he certainly wasn't congratulating us so much as bragging, Grandpa had finally showed us the hand. "We're smart?" I asked Pat.

Our parents were intelligent, too. Each was the only one of their siblings to finish high school. They both attended college briefly. Of course, not all of intelligence is rendered by genes. The odds are just as good you'll be less intelligent than your parents. We might have won the genetic toss-up, but having parents who helped with homework and projects was a real advantage. Neither of my parents grew up in homes where someone was available or able to help them with their studies.

There were times when we hadn't studied enough for a test or finished a project that our parents would let us stay home until we were prepared. They gave our education everything they had, and that made a huge difference. Pat was able to graduate from college, not a small feat for someone with schizophrenia. Onset in males is typically age eighteen to twenty-five— they hardly stand a chance. Pat received his degree in 2005, a year later than he would have had he studied straight through. He was almost twenty-four years old. Onset had begun years earlier and was particularly insidious. No one saw what was happening, so no one was helping him through his last year of college. It was a struggle, but he wrote and defended a thesis and graduated with honors.

My parents didn't talk about being proud of us. We would usually hear it through their friends: "He talks about you all the time" or "Your mother is so proud of you." They wanted us to be as modest as we were hardworking.

Something that separated me from my brother was that he seemed to belong in my family, whereas I did not. Despite my being overtly shy, my parents called me "Sarah Bernhardt" after the French actress. They said I was overly dramatic, reactive, and emotional. The nickname was a joke to them, but it made me think something was wrong with me.

Dad thought most of my school stories were tall tales. Mom never believed me when I claimed to be sick. I started to believe I didn't fit into my family. That's when I started writing. I figured if I wrote it down, someday someone would read it and believe me. When I didn't know how to write the words I wanted, I asked my mother to transcribe. I often dictated to her in the carpool line, waiting for Pat to get out of karate class.

Looking back, I was a typical little girl. I was expressive and sensitive. I didn't throw tantrums, I wasn't loud or obnoxious, and I was rarely the center of attention. My brother would have said I was overreactive, but he also couldn't deny that there were times when he shoved me into a closet with the lights out and held the door shut for over a minute. Like most little sisters I tattled, whined, and liked to be consoled. But there was something archaic and probably a little southern that cast me in a different light. Boys were considered princely, and girls were just sort of silly and hysterical. When I was active or expressive, it was often seen as obnoxious or defiant, whereas with Pat it was viewed as leadership. My brother was funny, whereas I was too sarcastic. Pat was sick, but I was faking it. Sleeping until noon on Saturday meant I was lazy, but Pat was just tired. There was a double standard. What made it worse was that I was nothing like my mother. I was rather tomboyish and androgynous, at least on the inside. Many people are surprised to learn that I always felt I was pretty terrible at being a girl.

I spent a great deal of time outdoors as a kid. For most of my life we lived in a house in the country with three acres of yard and a large pond full of catfish. I would come home from school, cut up some hotdogs, and use them to catch perch from the pond. I would take a pasta strainer from the house and use it to capture minnows. I played in the sprinklers and swam in the pond, even if it was too cold. When Dad was washing cars, I would run through the hose. Eventually I'd end up sitting in the soap bucket, because I fit in it. I liked fitting myself into things. Pat liked the water too. I remember vividly a creek behind our house overflowing after a storm. We got up Saturday morning in our pajamas and went kicking and stomping around in the muddy water for hours.

We lived in the country but went to school in a more suburban area. When I was little, it seemed like the best of both worlds. Kids came over, and I would take them on adventures all over the yard. Pat practiced several sports out there too. We had room for lots of pets, family gatherings, and exploration.

2

Growing Pains and Creative Outlets

If I had to put my finger on something that set us apart from other families, I would say it was our "communication deviance," a term I picked up in psychopathology class. Communication was broken, mired by feelings of inadequacy, anxiety, oversensitivity, absolutism, and perfectionism. Mom and Dad were constantly too hard on us. It's hard to communicate when you're afraid of being judged or seeming vulnerable, so what you mean to say gets mismanaged and comes out wrong. It's something that occurs throughout our extended family, passed down through the paternal line.

Our parents would talk *around* us, passing messages alone, and saying things to one another that they should have said to us. Praise was passed around but never met our ears, just like the standardized test scores. Often the things they told us were incomplete or vague. Lack of communication means you have to mind-read, interpret gestures, and listen carefully for tone shifts. It breeds paranoia. If all your relationships are like this, most of the things you would know about a person are just things you suspect.

We were spanked when we were little. The weird thing is that the only vivid memories I have of being spanked are the times I didn't know why it was happening. It wasn't until we were adults that Pat and I shared these memories. He remembered the same thing, not knowing what he had done wrong. It felt unfair, if not just senseless. It was like getting caught in the middle of something that had nothing to do with me. Perhaps the tensions in our parents' marriage were getting the best of them.

Even then you could see glimpses of our parents in us. Pat and I often beat ourselves up about things we had no control over. We are perfectionists. If we do something, we aim to do it perfectly. We don't like to talk to other people about how they make us feel. We have trouble apologizing, especially to someone's face. I always told myself it's because actions speak much louder than words, but I can't discount the possibility that I learned it from my parents.

I often found myself in friendships with other girls who were very controlling and possessive of me. I always had a best friend who didn't want to share me with anyone else. I never figured out why; maybe I was just too passive. On the other hand, Pat could be very controlling. We had a lot of dogs growing up, some still alive after all these years. Pat and I had different ways with them. I was extremely affectionate and tended to let them do whatever they wanted. I love seeing personality in a dog, watching it get a big idea and acting on it. It's fascinating and funny: "Look, he found a way to get onto the table!"

Pat was more energetic and playful, but also more controlling. Kurt Vonnegut always wrote about his love for dogs and how he would devote so much time to just playing with them. Pat was much the same. But when a dog won't listen to his command, it's as if it hurts his feelings. He seems disappointed, irritated, or maybe even embarrassed. When we were young, I'd find him sitting in the yard, with the dog nearby. Pat wouldn't even look at him. When I asked him what was going on, he'd say the dog wasn't listening to him. Pat needed time to recover from the disappointment.

I couldn't figure out exactly what it was that pleased our parents, although it was all I wanted. Nothing can describe the sweetness, the way praise emboldened our lost little minds. But while we were trying to adapt to this broken system, we weren't learning anything that would be useful to us in the world at large. I was remarkably socially awkward into adulthood. I had a pretty good idea how to make my parents happy, but I had no idea how to talk to my peers, especially the opposite sex.

I was thirteen when my cousin from Missouri came to visit us. She was a few months older than me. She was an outgoing, athletic blond girl with a sweet southern drawl. I had met her the year before during a family reunion. Somehow it seemed so much easier as a child to meet a new person, make friends, and do things together. At thirteen years old, I didn't know what to say. I didn't know how to welcome her to my house or how to ask her to do things with me. I was afraid of rejection and of looking stupid. I was so self-conscious that I ignored her for days. It became my thing. I had to keep acting like I didn't like her and didn't notice her when she walked into a room, or somehow the charade would be all for nothing and I'd look even more foolish. I even swam in the pool with her and pretended she wasn't there. Toward the end of her visit, something happened, probably just asking her to pass me something, and that's when we finally started talking. She was a really nice girl and made it easy to give up my stupid grudge.

My cousin was sad when I was ignoring her. As soon as I started talking to her she became happy. Just like that, she forgave me and was satisfied. I wondered why I wasn't that way. I had trouble recovering from social faux pas, replaying them over and over again in my head. When she left, I beat myself up about how strangely I had behaved, but Pat said it wasn't a big deal because I did the right thing in the end.

Pat wasn't socially awkward when we were young. I joke that he learned it from me. He slowly became an introvert, a disposition that doesn't naturally change. It was all part of the little changes that took place for six years leading up to the diagnosis. They call that type of onset *insidious*. I can't think of any better name for it than that. It was so slow no one noticed, not until he was sick.

I was good at stifling myself and stamping out my desires. I never just said out loud, "Hey, I'm an idiot and I act weird sometimes. Can we still be friends?" There are a million situations where I didn't say what I wanted or meant, hid my true feelings, and just didn't act. Everyone has them, but I had many. And I regret them all.

At school, no one would have guessed that my nickname was "Sarah Bernhardt." As I grew older, I crawled firmly into my shell and didn't even come out in private. Meanwhile, Pat had popular girls calling him at home. If he missed a day of school, almost his entire grade would ask me if he was okay. His arm was broken when he was thirteen. While playing basketball at a friend's house, he slipped on a sheet of algae in the driveway. All his weight went down, crushing his left elbow. It had to be rebuilt with eighteen screws, ten pins, and four plates. I remember it well because it was my eleventh birthday. In fact, young and ignorant, I was actually mad at him for making me spend my birthday in the hospital. I wasn't really mad that he had changed my birthday plans. I was just jealous.

Things seemed to come so easily to Pat. Kids at school loved his cast, loved his resilience, and even loved the long scar it left. He had physical therapy every week for months, and as much as it hurt him, he faced it without any whining or complaining. The therapist would pull down on his hand, and he was supposed to pull back up. I remember him gritting his teeth and the tears welling up in his eyes when he would bear down. When they let go, he just gasped and regained his composure.

He matured faster than other kids. He was taller and hairier than the average thirteen-year-old. He was very independent, and that frightened me. I could catch up intellectually, but I was afraid of new things and novel situations. I didn't like talking to strangers. I wouldn't even make my own doctor's appointments. Pat took readily to new responsibilities. He couldn't wait to drive himself everywhere. He didn't want to do things with the family. He would walk ahead of us when we went to the mall, like he wasn't with us. My parents saw this as healthy. "He's becoming a young man," they said. Pat wanted to run his own errands, do his own laundry, have his own account at the video store, and pay his own late fees.

Meanwhile, I rarely accepted invites to parties. Eventually I stopped getting them. I kept journals and wrote poetry, despite a great deal of mocking from my brother. I read horror novels and watched forensic reality television shows. I listened to music that was unpopular for my age group, particularly classic rock. I couldn't help that the things I liked weren't popular, and I grew to believe that I was just smarter than everyone else. My room was covered in posters: the Beatles, Jimi Hendrix, *A Clockwork Orange*. I would burn incense every night. When my dad would knock on my door, he'd say he felt like he had stepped back in time. I loved that.

My grades in math started to slip. They would only get worse as I got older. It was like I just couldn't process the information the way my classmates could. I spent hours every night doing my math homework, checking my answers, and then doing them again. Most students didn't *study* for math tests in fifth grade, but I had to. It helped nothing. My grades didn't reflect the effort I put in at all. People didn't seem to know how to help me. Friends and teachers would watch me work through a problem and just seem baffled, like I was a malfunctioning computer. Pat would try to help me, but for him, getting the right answer was as simple as just doing the work.

When I took geometry in ninth grade, my dad went to my school for parent-teacher night. He showed my math teacher my report card: all As, except for a D in geometry. He said, "Now you can't tell me it's her. With grades like these, I know she's doing the work. It has to be you."

Soon sciences that included math—physics, chemistry—would be a problem for me too. But I was a shining star in art class. I was queen of English and literature. History was no problem. This disparity would indicate a learning disability. Of course, people don't like to throw that label around because it's misunderstood, just like everything else in the *DSM* (*Diagnostic and Statistical Manual of Mental Disorders*).

Put simply, I couldn't learn mathematics using the same methods as my classmates. In another country, in a different school system, using different books, and maybe with a more creative perspective on getting to the right answer, I might not have struggled to pass mathematics. Personally it feels better to know that something was going on that wasn't under my control. After years of math homework, tutors, spending the majority of my time working and reworking problems, success just wasn't in the cards. My poor teachers saw me working so hard they made sure to pass me. Still I could never tackle it. All I could do was bury my head.

Pat and I were always extremely creative. Pat played the guitar, just like Dad, which always made me feel like I had lost a contest. I painted, wrote, and drew. I could create almost anything with my hands, but not music. I hated the practice, the endless repetition until I finally got it right. I felt it took too long.

Dad showed Pat how to play the intro of Ozzy Osbourne's "Crazy Train" when he was twelve. Dad went to mow the lawn and left Pat to practice. By the afternoon, he was playing it with such proficiency that when Dad came inside he thought Pat had put on his old vinyl album. He had a creative knack for the guitar that was uncanny. Barely a teen, he was writing songs and reaching a level of technical ability that many guitarists never achieve.

Our paths were becoming very clear. I would be an artist, a writer. Pat would be a guitarist, a lover of big ideas, and maybe even a teacher.

Was there anything about Pat as a child that indicated he would be diagnosed with paranoid schizophrenia when he was twenty-five? No. He never behaved strangely or frightened me. He was very reasonable. Actually, he was the person a lot of people went to for advice. Emotionally he was usually on an even keel. He never did anything to make me truly fear him. He wasn't skeptical or sarcastic until we were teenagers. He got along well with just about everyone.

Sitting in a graduate-level psychology course, a fellow student who worked in social services for years commented that schizophrenics have terrible family histories. It made me feel ashamed that someone would go spreading around a lie like that. We may have been dysfunctional, but there were no horrors in our past. The world is full of dysfunctional families, ranging from comical to criminal, and the vast majority of children in those families do not have schizophrenia. In fact, schizophrenia only occurs in about 1 percent of the population, while family dysfunction is so common it's almost the norm. We weren't perfect, but the beautiful thing about our family is that we learn from our mistakes. We change and grow all the time. How many families can match that?

What in our past, if anything, could have predicted that Pat would develop schizophrenia? I read a study where scientists went looking for evidence in videos taken when patients were only children.[1] Researchers gathered home movies featuring patients who experienced adult-onset schizophrenia and their healthy siblings. The children were only eight years old or younger in the home movies. In every case the sibling with schizophrenia was the only person in their immediate family with a psychiatric disease. The footage was edited so that there were only scenes of one or more of the children, with no cuts to grandma or the family dog. Then the chronologically ordered segments were shown to graduate students. Blind to the psychiatric status of the siblings in the film, the students had to identify which one of the children would later develop schizophrenia. Far above chance, the students most often correctly identified the sibling with adult-onset schizophrenia. The kid was just different somehow, not ordinary. The results have stood as primary evidence that through observed behavior we can see the makings of schizophrenia; processes are at work in childhood even though onset may not occur until adulthood. It's not to be misconstrued as a discovery that will predict schizophrenia, but rather as evidence of early *vulnerabilities* that could put one at risk for a variety of disorders including schizophrenia.

Pat and I would have fit perfectly into the sample they used. When I read the study, I immediately thought of a home movie of Pat and me opening Christmas presents in 1989. Originally from northeast Arkansas, our mom still had her country accent. She sat on the floor with us, picking up empty packaging and feigning excitement with each gift we opened. Dad was behind the camera. Pat had just found a present hidden in the dining room. Just like in *A Christmas Story*, it was a BB gun. He was so happy he could hardly talk. I stood over him in my nightgown, a big T-shirt, saying, "Wow, Pat! Whoa! Wow! Oh, that's so cool." I was awkwardly trying to be a part of his surprise while simultaneously hiding the fact that I was hurt I didn't get a surprise too. I was partly trying to work out if this BB gun was also for me, but I could plainly see that the label said "Pat." He took it out of the box and held it up so he could look through the sight on top. I stood over him for long minutes just repeating myself, "Whoa, cool." Which one of us would they have found *unusual* in that video? What did no one see when we were children?

3

Hurtful Family Ties

Mom is from Arkansas. All her family live there, so they didn't play a huge part in our lives growing up in New Orleans. Her mother would come for visits, usually during holidays, but most of our family get-togethers consisted of just Dad's family. One particular holiday comes to mind now: Father's Day in 1996. My grandmother, Maw-Maw Alice, had us over for lunch. As it was a surprisingly cool summer day, my Uncle Larry, Dad, Pat, and I helped to set up a table on the back porch so we could eat outside. My mom was out of town in Arkansas, maybe for a funeral. There were many important gatherings on her side of the family that we kids missed for some reason.

Maw-Maw Alice and Grandpa Howard have been separated for as long as I can remember. I was the only kid in my grade whose grandparents weren't together. It raised a lot of questions with other kids when they took turns picking me up from school in the afternoon. "No, they're not divorced, just separated." As I grew up, I began to understand the situation more and more. Alice wanted a divorce and Howard didn't. So they worked out a financial agreement. They lived separately; he gave her a small monthly stipend as spending money and he paid for all big-ticket items like houses, cars, and vacations. This way Howard kept all the money and doled it out as he saw fit. I'm not sure why Alice agreed to this.

That Father's Day, we were sitting on the patio eating in the shade when Maw-Maw started talking about her brother Earl. I didn't know many of her siblings. Most lived in other cities, and others had died before I was born. She was always telling me that Uncle Tom was like this or Aunt Audrey liked to do that. Uncle Earl had been mildly mentally retarded and an alcoholic. He died young, and it was very painful for her. But today, at the sheer mention of the name "Earl," Grandpa flew into a rage. It came from nowhere. There was no warning. "Earl was a rotten piece of shit just like the rest of your goddamn family."

Maw-Maw's mouth hung open. I was stunned. It reminded me of something I'd seen on a TV show: a kid involuntarily shouting obscenities in a shopping mall. Was this Tourette syndrome?

"Earl was a good m—"

Howard interrupted: "He was a good-for-nothing, piece-of-shit asshole. What do you know, you stupid cunt?" This was the first time I had ever heard the C-word used in real life. I was twelve years old.

Pat and I sat in shock, glancing at each other nervously. We knew our grandfather had a temper, but we never saw him act this way. Until then, I'd only ever seen him have an outburst in traffic.

Grandpa got up and threw his napkin on the table. He was red faced and breathing heavily. He kept muttering bad names at Maw-Maw. It made no sense to me. As far as I could tell, she hadn't insulted him or even mentioned Grandpa. It was almost as if he flew into a rage because she was talking at all. Had he heard what she said or imagined she was implying something else?

Maw-Maw picked at her food and mumbled. The fact that she wasn't intimidated by his rage might have made it worse. A big, heavy man looming over a tiny lady, yet she deflected his hostility rather easily. I guess there wasn't much to fear but the spit flying from his mouth as he cursed.

After yelling at Maw-Maw, he stomped inside in his slow, lumbering way. Then he was gone. Presumably he went home. Probably to a bar, Dad said. Pat and I had never seen a fight like that before. Maw-Maw kept protesting to herself, "Earl was a good man." Dad and Uncle Larry wanted her to shut up. Surely this was something they had seen play out in their household over and over growing up. And finally I saw it for myself. If someone had said those things to my mother, I would have stuck up for her and asked them to leave. But this was different. Dad and Larry had to bear the beast growing up, and Maw-Maw never flew to their defense.

I couldn't wait to tell Mom about what had happened that day. I was sure she wouldn't be able to believe it. I was wrong. She said, "If Grandpa is perfectly comfortable losing his cool in front of us now, he'll be doing it more often from now on." I asked what she meant. "You're all grown up now. He's not going to make an effort to hide it anymore."

Of course Grandpa's tantrum didn't happen until he finished his meal. From then on, I noticed this trend. He got a plate of food first and finished it almost as soon as everyone was seated. He waited until he'd had a second helping and then sat back watching us all. Then he'd try to pick a fight. He'd say anything to get a rise out of someone, and if it didn't work, he'd move on to the next person. He liked to needle Maw-Maw by calling her the wrong name. "You got enough turkey, Alexis? Alexis, you made that oyster stuffing?" But then Maw-Maw Alice was the least "fun" because she never seemed unsettled. She usually just rolled her eyes. Grandpa would turn to someone else, "Remember that time you broke your grandmother's punch bowl at her birthday party?"

Grandpa didn't like to be argued with and considered people who did to be "ungrateful." But the best holidays ended in arguments. Grandpa would get up from the table, storm out of the house, and then we were all free to finally enjoy ourselves. We had second helpings and another glass of wine because he wasn't there to call anyone "fatso" or "stupid drunk."

Usually he didn't curse. That kind of language was saved for Maw-Maw. He never backed down from a brawl, though. My dad and Uncle Larry used to tell me stories about fights he got into at bars, even in his old age. One Christmas Eve, he got in a cousin's face, as if to fight him. Grandpa was seventy at the time, and my cousin was thirty-five years old. No one is really sure what he was angry about. As usual, it seemed to come out of nowhere.

Before I was twelve, I thought the stories of Grandpa's rage were exaggerated. I would go to Maw-Maw's house and find I had just missed him. She would tell me, "Your Grandpa just stormed out of here." But I took it with a grain of salt. I heard about the way he treated his kids—beating them with belts, throwing things at them. He taunted my Uncle Larry for being a heavy kid, hiding behind the refrigerator, waiting for him to open it, and then jumping out from behind it shouting, "You're fat! Fatso!" I never saw him do anything quite so vindictive, so it seemed to me he must have mellowed. I was wrong; I was just too young to notice.

Dad and Larry were five years apart in age. As kids, they ate dinner before Grandpa got home from work so they didn't have to hear his jibes about Dad's acne or Larry's weight. If these comments didn't upset them, he would try harder, getting onto them about just about anything. Once they stopped having family meals, Grandpa started eating in his bedroom with the door shut. Maw-Maw would wait on him hand and foot so he never had to get up unless he needed to use the bathroom. He used an actual overbed table from a hospital so he could eat lying down.

As teenagers, Dad and Larry wouldn't come home at night until they knew he was asleep. My uncle slept out on the patio furniture, getting eaten by mosquitoes one night because Grandpa stayed up unusually late. Both sons left home before they were eighteen.

They walked around on eggshells, never knowing what their dad would do next. It took nothing to set him off. He would find strange ways to debase and humiliate them. When my dad was sixteen, my grandfather told him to go into the living room and show his houseguests his pimples. Grandpa pretended this was all in good humor. Dad refused; he was the only one to ever fight back. Grandpa flew into a rage and threw a heavy marble ashtray across the room at him. It smashed against the wall and crumbled to the floor. After that, Dad moved out of the family home and in with an aunt. Dad finished high school with an award for never missing a day of school. Anyone could have guessed why. I can only wonder what could have been if he had left Grandpa's home sooner.

I was never afraid of Grandpa Howard. He picked Pat and me up from elementary school three days a week. It was the only time that Pat told me to sit in the front seat; he had no interest in riding shotgun. Grandpa would take us to his apartment, which was always dirty and completely devoid of food. There were some cans of green beans, a box of stale cereal that I had picked the raisins out of six months ago, and moldy mayonnaise. To prove that Grandpa never bothered with his kitchen, one day we put a rock in his freezer. He never mentioned it, so I assume he never found it. Sometime in our twenties, Pat went into his freezer and retrieved the rock. We kept it. It was important to us for some reason to rescue it from that place.

His one-bedroom apartment had two televisions; otherwise there were just dusty newspapers, empty bookshelves, and half-finished crossword puzzles. I remember it smelled of mildew and oily scalp. After school, he'd drop us off, usually not coming into the apartment at all. He was on his way to happy hour. We'd wait there until our parents finished work several hours later. It was miserable and boring. It was worse for Pat. We were always hungry when we left school. Pat was overweight, and Grandpa would take any opportunity to point it out. There's a rumor in the family that when Pat was still in kindergarten, Grandpa threatened to call child services on my parents because Pat was fat. He claimed our parents must be force-feeding him.

Some days Grandpa would buy us food, but he had to dictate what we ate. We could eat grilled chicken sandwiches from fast-food restaurants, but no burgers, fries, or sodas. He would get himself a double cheeseburger. We could have ice cream, but only if he was in the mood for it, too. If he took us to school in the morning, he'd let Pat get a breakfast sandwich and I could have a hash brown, but he would have a deluxe breakfast himself, with pancakes, eggs, and sausage. He would tell me to eat faster and Pat to eat slower. He always said, "You're wolfing it, Pat!"

Other days, I would get into his car and see empty cans of soda and candy bar wrappers. He had stopped at a gas station on his way to pick us up. That meant he'd already eaten, so he wasn't going to stop and get us anything.

He was obsessed with other people's eating habits and weight, but for as long as I can remember, Grandpa himself was very heavy and unenergetic. He was tall and unwieldy. He always moved slowly, taking tiny steps and breathing heavily. He seemed to be much older than his years, always moaning about aches and pains. He would have a coughing fit, but apparently he had perfectly healthy lungs. In fact, he had no physical ailments to speak of. Yet he always asked people to help him out of chairs and into cars. A hypochondriac, he saw the doctor for simple indigestion or sore muscles. Despite being overweight, his stress tests were always good. I'm sure that disappointed him. At sixty, it took him five minutes to mount one flight of stairs. And he made a big show of it, huffing and puffing, groaning, and saying things like, "Oh, Holy Mary." I remember he would never help me carry my schoolbag. He never carried anything.

He used to tell me I was out of control and wild. He was referring to me singing and swinging my legs all the way home from school. It was an exaggeration. I knew enough kids to know I was a good one. I would come home from school with treats for good behavior, and he would ask, "How come you're so good in school and so bad when I pick you up?" I told him that I had to be bad *sometime*. It was nice to be thin, and it was nice to not care what Grandpa said. It was nice to be a girl. Grandpa seemed to hate males the most. He took great pride in making Pat angry by needling him about his weight. He would berate my younger cousin Sean, too, and tell him he would be a loser just like his father.

He didn't talk to me about anything unless he was fishing for something to make fun of. He asked about grades and if I'd made any friends that day. He would ask me how often I cleaned my fingernails, picking up my hands and looking disgusted. If I bit my nails, he'd grab my hand and say, "Ugh, getting those dirty nails in your mouth?" He'd crack my knuckles without so much as a warning, and I'd let out a gasp and pull my hand away.

Being around him didn't make puberty any easier. He'd ask how many Cokes I drank because that was why I had so many pimples. He wanted to know if there was some way to straighten my hair or if I wanted braces for my teeth. I would roll my eyes and fall into silence. At least he had no control over my life whatsoever. That was what made him bearable. He sat in judgment of everything I said and did, but in the end nothing he said mattered to anyone.

I know when Grandpa is judging someone inferior because he smiles as he speaks. If he truly likes something, it will render him speechless. But if he's grinning and talking, he's thinking terrible things about you on the inside, probably something petty. The smile is the definition of smug. The inferiority of others amuses him. Few people have ever intimidated him. Usually they were accomplished people who had something he wanted. There was only one time I saw him speechless. I had a friend in high school who won awards for her harp and piano performances. Once she opened for the Louisiana Philharmonic. When my grandfather met her, he actually blushed.

But no matter what, he always had a short fuse. He would yell at other cars in traffic, nearly climbing onto the dashboard to shout, "What the hell are you doing, you goddamn idiot?" He'd get so loud that my ears would ring. I always wondered, does he think they can hear him?

He also liked to talk trash. He managed to tell us on a weekly basis, "Your Dad's an asshole."

Pat would be furious. He was that boy who always told his friends, "My Dad says . . . ."

Grandpa would say, "I bet your no-good, son-of-a-bitch Dad taught you that!" Then they would argue all the way to the apartment. Pat would be in a funk, and Grandpa would just drive off to happy hour like he didn't miss a beat. I think he took energy from putting people down. Hurt feelings were like snacks to him.

I was about ten years old the first time he told me to handle his funeral arrangements. I don't know why Grandpa didn't ask his wife or sons to carry out his wishes. He said he wanted to be cremated, and he wanted me to keep the ashes. Over time his wishes got more elaborate. He said I should put some of the ashes in a potted plant and care for it so it grew strong and tall. Then he wanted me to put some of the ashes on my forehead when I got married, so he could be there for the ceremony even after he died. My parents were shocked when I told them—not just because it was an inappropriately morbid thing to say to a ten-year-old, or the fact that Grandpa was in good health, but because I wasn't even close with him.

Looking back, I don't think he asked this of me because he thought we were close. He did it because he thought I was submissive enough to follow his wishes, that I would do what he said without question, and because my sense of obligation would keep me true. I never fought him outright, and that to him meant I respected him. But I knew as a child, when he told me his wishes, that I would not be putting him on my forehead. Since then, he's passed the duty of his funeral arrangements to my younger cousins, who feel quite the same as I did.

Some days, Grandpa was oddly energetic and goofy, singing show tunes, usually *West Side Story*, or just generally singing something he was think-ing about. When I was very young he would sing an old song called "Buckle Down, Winsocki," and that was my cue to put my seat belt on. He taught me the lyrics and we'd sing it together. Pat sat in the backseat ignoring us. After the siege at Waco in 1993, he made up a song by rhyming anything he could with "Branch Davidian." I thought it was funny, but that sort of thing only made Pat really angry. Beasts can't be cute. It's hard to imagine that someone who liked singing show tunes could also have such an explosive temper.

Those crazy, quirky things that Grandpa did made sense to me. As far as I knew, he was kooky. All my life he called me "Sarah Kate." I always thought it was a reference to something else, maybe a character from an old TV show or a musical. I was in high school before I learned that he thought Kate was my middle name. God knows why. No one had ever corrected him because they just thought he was being kooky. Obviously other people didn't take him seriously either. I wish Pat had been one of those people. It took him a long time to cool off after an argument with Grandpa. He never asked me why I didn't argue with him too. Pat thought it was his job to make the arguments, to stand defense. He often assumed the role of parent when it was just the two of us alone.

After Grandpa would drop us off, I was excited to have the time to my-self. Pat was just frustrated. He was trying to crack the code, to find the thing to say that would finally make him shut up, without using the cursing and name-calling that Grandpa employed. It wasn't fair. A kid shouldn't have to argue with an adult, let alone hear his father talked about that way. We did tell our parents about these incidents, but they brushed it off. It wasn't anything new to them.

We loved the days that Maw-Maw picked us up from school. She always gave us food, whatever we liked—it was our choice. She'd even have dinner waiting when our parents got off work. Being with Maw-Maw was being on completely neutral ground. She loved kids. If there were toddlers in her house, you'd always find her on the floor with them. We didn't have to be perfect with her. We could just be kids. She kept Chef Boyardee and frozen chicken nuggets in her fridge, things she knew kids liked to eat. She let us watch scary movies and swear. She was my only relative that I was proud to introduce to my friends. I knew they would love her as much as I did. "This is my Maw-Maw. She has the highest score on Pac-Man that you've ever seen in your life."

I could tell her how I felt about things without feeling judged obnoxious or overly emotional. I was about twelve when I went to eat dinner with her, Grandpa, and my aunt and uncle. I noticed that the men spent all night talking to each other, while the women at the table spent the evening in relative silence. I think the only thing my aunt or Maw-Maw said all night was something about the bread and about the soup they ordered. On the way home, alone in the van with Maw-Maw, I started crying. I asked her why we sat there silently all night, just watching the men talk. At first it seemed as if she hadn't even noticed. Then she said, "Sarah, I'm really impressed you noticed that. It shouldn't be like that. You're right." Just hearing that was all I needed. It made me feel normal.

As awful as Grandpa Howard could be, I think having a little Alice in us might be our saving grace. At some point, I think all of the grandkids had a moment when we wished we could stay at Maw-Maw's forever. Maybe that's just because she would have let us stay home from school. She would have even done our homework for us like she had with Aunt Sue. Maw-Maw let us be ourselves. That was the most important thing. We could relax with her and be imperfect.

4

Breaking Free

Grandpa owned a real estate agency where Dad and my Uncle Larry worked. Dad started working for Grandpa when he was about twenty. He left college and decided he would get some certifications in real estate. At some point both Dad and Uncle Larry were fired from the agency, Larry repeatedly. Grandpa would get mad at them for something non-work-related; then he would verbally debase them in front of their coworkers and send them packing. I was only a baby at the time. With a newborn at home, my dad just decided he wouldn't accept it. He went into work the next day like nothing had ever happened, and Grandpa never said anything. Uncle Larry, on the other hand, was out of work sometimes for almost a year before Maw-Maw Alice would convince Grandpa to hire him back. Larry also had three small children at home.

Our parents shrugged off the spats between Pat and Grandpa. Given that Grandpa was prone to fire people at the slightest sign of insubordination, Dad was in no position to confront him about it. Instead our parents said that we were mature enough to handle ourselves, and to know not to put any stock in what the old man said. Pat didn't understand why he had to conduct himself in a mature manner if Grandpa didn't. He couldn't wait until he was old enough to drive so he could take us to and from school himself.

Grandpa wasn't the only source of family dysfunction. We often found out how a relative really felt through gossip. Despite having been complimentary to his face, Pat would learn that our cousin thought his girlfriend was "funny looking" from Uncle Larry. Pat would fume for a moment and get a little red faced. Then he'd respond, "Whatever," and drop the subject. I'm not sure if the anger he felt was gone or if he had buried it deep down.

"Don't ever let them get a reaction out of you," he told me once. "That's what they want." I'm not sure if that's what they intended, but it seemed like the only reasonable explanation. I have never enjoyed watching someone lose their cool, but then I would never disparage their girlfriend either.

It was hard to work out the point of being close with one's family when ours was generally rude and unsupportive. Rather than being proud of us, they could become strangely competitive. Aunt Sue was twenty years older than me and once wanted to be an actress. After I was cast as the lead in a seventh-grade school play, she would always bring up the fact that during the performance I had a big bruise on my shin, which the whole audience could see.

"What's that got to do with anything?" Pat would ask.

"Nothing. I just thought someone would have touched it up. Wasn't there anyone to do your makeup, Sarah?" she asked, sipping a glass of wine.

"I guess not," I said. I tried to take her comments with a grain of salt, but I wanted to cry. Rather than remembering the compliments I got on my performance, more often I just remember the bruise.

Conversations like this added a great deal of tension to family relations. Criticism often hid just below the surface of what they said. If someone congratulated Pat on making the honor roll, I would worry about what they were really saying about him behind his back. I felt I could never trust what they said. Our father told us, "Don't listen to them; they're just jealous."

Dad's family also liked to stir the pot. After two relatives had an argument, their phones would ring off the hook. Everyone wanted to hear each version of the story, and they would spread it like wildfire. Of course, just like a game of telephone, the end result would be some strange distortion of the actual event, and tempers would flare up all over again when it reached the source.

I learned from Pat to behave differently around our relatives. I didn't disclose much, and I kept conversations on a superficial level. Sometimes I would be rude and standoffish rather than let slip something close to my heart. I found it difficult and upsetting. It was easier for me to just avoid family altogether. Pat didn't mind shape-shifting each time we saw our relatives. While he was more open and funny with his friends, he never shared anything too deep with them either. For Pat, time with his friends was an opportunity to escape from the hypercritical environment of family and the grueling discipline of school. He didn't tell other people about the things that went on with Grandpa or the rest of the family, as if he thought that would muck up his healthy relationships.

I admired the way Pat could separate reality from the hypercritical comments our family made. But he was still affected by the things they said. It definitely multiplied the self-consciousness that comes with puberty. When we reached high school, Pat was often on crash diets. Sometimes I would hear him in the bathroom purging dinner. He tried weight training and diet pills to no avail. He would lose twenty pounds and in several months gain thirty. He would buy new, smaller clothes and not fit into them nine months later. He would not get a handle on his weight until college, at which point his illness was taking hold.

Embarrassment kept us from bringing a lot of new people around our relatives. Many friends of the family were lost after something inappropriate happened, usually the minute they heard Grandpa howl and curse. It created a clannish environment. Not only were new people given the cold shoulder, but new ideas were also shut out. A common sentiment around the dinner table at family gatherings was utmost skepticism for anything new. Whether someone had read a book or seen something on TV, it was scoffed at. Subjects like science could be particularly prickly.

While my parents seemed to think that family spats were a part of life, all my experiences were telling me otherwise. My friends felt affection for their grandfathers and looked forward to spending time with them. Their unhappy grandparents or parents got divorced and usually worked hard to keep the peace in front of the kids. Their families were proud of them and talked about their accomplishments.

Part of me wanted to tell my friends, "Guess what screwed up thing happened at my house on Easter," but I kept it to myself. The older I got the more contrast there was between my family and others'. I didn't want anyone to know what kind I came from. I was afraid my friends would revoke my normal person's license if they saw behind the curtain. I worked so hard to be different, to be positive, insightful, compassionate, and open-minded. I didn't want my family to blow it for me. Despite what you see in comedies, dysfunctional families don't make good anecdotes.

My friends felt true happiness for me when I accomplished something. When I confided in them, they didn't spread ugly rumors about me. It made sense if other kids were competitive with me because they were my peers. The world at large didn't appear to be two-faced. In fact, it seemed to be mostly straightforward and genuine. This was contrary to how I felt around my relatives.

To be fair, the kind of upbringing we went through had nothing to do with where we grew up. I don't know any other families like ours. I'm not sure growing up in Arkansas would have been much better. Mom is from a small town where people spend most of their time gossiping. Nothing is private. Everyone knows everyone else, at least to the degree that they feel comfortable spreading rumors about them. That kind of environment is also rife with paranoia.

As we got older we saw our extended family less and less. It was only natural as we entered our teens, but it was also linked to the fact that Mom started working again. Our nuclear family was more financially independent and didn't have to worry about walking on eggshells to please Grandpa. We began having holiday dinners to ourselves, just the four of us. It could be a little lonely, often too quiet to feel like a holiday. But Pat and I never saw any more explosive arguments. No one got drunk and had to go home in a cab. No one criticized Pat's eating habits or my unclear skin.

Dad still worked with Grandpa every day. His proficiency at selling homes was growing, and his job was more secure because of it. Suddenly the agency was getting bigger and bigger. I can remember when my family started making more money, because we suddenly bought much more food each time we went to the grocery store. We finally did things like shop for back-to-school clothes and got Christmas presents for my teachers. We got our first computer in 1997. Looking back, though, I have to wonder why it took so long. Dad had been working there since the 1970s. I wonder how long it took before his commission was increased.

It seemed that Grandpa resented Dad even more after he was successful. Maybe he felt threatened by his sons. He had no intention of retiring, though he never went into the office anymore. When he did go in, there was a concert of ringing phones, with people calling each other to warn them that he was there. He usually just went in to chitchat with people or to talk to Dad about finances. He would complain about money, family, and politics. Trying to get work done without snubbing him, the staff was a captive audience. They would learn about his aches and pains or about a fight he had gotten into. Sometimes a secretary would accompany him to a grandkid's school play.

Pat and I began working at the agency after high school. Our jobs were a direct result of something Grandpa had done. He had hired a broker named Analee, who left the agency to go into business for herself. The problem was that she was in breach of the noncompete clause in her contract. She even tried to take some accounts with her. Pat and I were tasked with sending out mailers to fix the mass confusion it created among clients.

The strange thing was that Grandpa and Analee had been good friends. She may have been his only friend. They went nearly everywhere together. In eighth grade, he brought her to my graduation. Maw-Maw used to complain to me that she thought they were having an affair, but it seemed platonic to me. Then suddenly Analee didn't even want to talk to Grandpa. When asked why, he played dumb about the new schism between them. Everyone was at a loss as to what had changed.

The agency sued her for breach of contract; then she filed suit for sexual harassment against Grandpa. Everything was coming to pieces. Instead of being forthcoming so that maybe we could help, Grandpa remained tight-lipped. Then something happened that turned the tide. At some point Dad got a voice mail from a private number. A man's voice that he did not recognize accused him of being a selfish "sociopath" and of hurting anyone who got in his way. The phone records were subpoenaed, and it turned out to be a phone number belonging to Analee. She then suddenly dropped her sexual harassment suit.

Litigation went on for two years before they reached a settlement. Eventually attorneys would tease out what had happened between Grandpa and Analee. He had brought her on as a broker, promising her that they would downsize and eventually run the business together. When he failed to make good with his side of the bargain, she quit. So, obviously Grandpa wanted his family out of the business.

It wasn't until this time that I realized that Pat always thought he would take over the agency. One evening we stopped by to visit with Maw-Maw Alice and found Grandpa there. He called to Pat from the spare bedroom. Reclining on the bed with his pants unbuckled and a remote control in his hand, he told Pat that he had never imagined he would go into real estate. Pat didn't get the impression that Grandpa thought he could "do so much more." He simply never saw Pat working in that area. Pat didn't ask what he saw him doing instead. In fact, he felt that it was a slight. Grandpa was telling him that he wasn't suited for working in the business, as if he was a lesser man than his father or his grandfather before him.

We smoked cigarettes on the back porch, and Pat shook off the conversation easily. "He just means you're smart—way smarter than you need to be if you're going to work at the agency."

"Run the agency," he corrected me.

"You don't need a bachelor's degree to run the agency. None of them went to college."

"But it's helpful."

I shrugged. "A business degree would be helpful. A philosophy degree is superfluous."

He rolled his eyes. "Trust me, Grandpa didn't mean it as a compliment."

"It doesn't matter. It's still a fact."

It seemed to me that we went to college to do something else. Surely we didn't need degrees if we were going into the family business. But that was exactly what Pat intended. Actually, he said he always felt it was expected of him. He didn't remember anyone explicitly telling him so, but he thought that as the heir apparent the job would fall to him. When he told me this, it was a startling glimpse into what Pat thought the future looked like. He was twenty-one, and despite studying philosophy in college, he would work in real estate. Whether or not he wanted to, he didn't say. It seemed to me to be a large sacrifice, a big leap, but for Pat it was just a given, just like when we were kids and he would assume the role of father when our parents weren't around. He always had a sense that all of Dad's responsibilities would one day be his. His future was spelled out for him. Meanwhile, I never imagined my life taking any course in particular. I never even imagined going to college, until I was there.

One thing was clear to me. My extended family had caused me a lot of pain and stress. I wanted to get away, and becoming an adult meant breaking free from them. I was one of the oldest grandkids, and I did worry for the others growing up in our family. But I couldn't take responsibility. My friends, parents, and brother were my sanctuary. I didn't need to have any idea where I was going in life, only that they were behind me. I didn't feel that they had any specific expectations of me, simply that I find happiness.

The diathesis-stress theory of schizophrenia posits that genetic predisposition combined with environmental stressors leads to the development of the disease. The way in which a person copes with stress can be healthy or unhealthy, reactive or proactive. Growing up I marveled at how well Pat could swallow unfairness, especially those times when he'd get in trouble and our parents just wouldn't listen to excuses. I could never let it go, but he seemed to accept it easily. He withdrew from the poisonous side of the family, while I stuck around, hoping they would change but continually getting hurt. He just accepted how it was. He didn't get emotionally wrapped up in things the way I did. Some people might call that "being a real man." But I wouldn't agree.

Today, I look at it differently. I don't marvel at his Zen-like acceptance. I see it for what it is: a history of avoidance of self-reflection. Pat didn't think very often about who he was and what he wanted out of life. His career and responsibilities were simply spelled out for him. He didn't think of himself as an autonomous being, but rather as someone who would inherit the responsibilities and life goals of others. He was an automaton. He just ignored most things he didn't like or couldn't change. If it ever came up, he'd bury it again, maybe this time with alcohol or marijuana. It's incredible how closely avoidance can resemble coping. Until the onset of his illness, I never saw him truly self-reflect.

5

His Sister's Keeper

You know that game where you name the first street you lived on and your biggest fear and together they make your "rock star name"? Mine would be Ponchatoula Failure. The game is much funnier if you lived on Interstate 80 Service Road West and are afraid of tarantulas. I'm not sure what Pat was most afraid of, but it was probably something more objective like losing his arms or legs. For me, fear of failure was the driving force for everything I did.

Eventually I got very good at beating myself up about perceived shortcomings. Even if I did something right, I would chastise myself for doing it too slowly or too awkwardly, and I certainly never gave myself any praise. I'd just move on to the next goal: "Okay, now you have to make an A on your research paper. You have to lose five pounds before Amanda's birthday party. Don't look at Zach when you walk into English. Get a pair of those boots all the other girls have."

I attended a small co-ed elementary school. While I was friends with nearly everyone, I easily overlooked that fact. I wanted a friend who really understood me, someone just like me. I liked to write poetry, read J. D. Salinger, listen to the Beatles and the Rolling Stones, burn incense, and stargaze. I watched horror movies every weekend. The only contemporary music I listened to was Marilyn Manson. It was a tall order. Feeling outcast, my daily attitude was somewhere in between sarcastic and brooding.

I was twelve years old when I first attempted suicide. It's hard to reveal this here and now, primarily because I'm at a loss to describe precisely how I felt back then. I don't usually talk to people about it now; it's more of a black hole in my personal history, something I can neither fully explain nor choose to pick at. However, rather than pass myself off as a perfect sister next to my somehow "imperfect" brother, I think it's important to uncover the things we have in common, the frustrations we may both have felt growing up. Besides, without Pat, I might never have gotten through it.

I suppose the overall feeling was that I was unwanted and no good to anyone. I had a magnifying glass over my flaws. A pimple made me a monster. If someone didn't compliment my outfit, it meant I looked awful. I couldn't find a friend who was very much like me because I was a ridiculous person, disgusting and put together all wrong. My grades in math meant I was an idiot. I was certain I was of no use to anyone and often a burden to all.

I had stopped growing and was realizing that I was a short person. I had acne and no boyfriend. It all felt insurmountable. My hair became very curly, almost unmanageable. I overheard my parents one evening having a conversation about it: "What should we do about Sarah's hair?" It was the same way people discuss telling a friend that they're worried about them. I didn't know kinky hair was an issue that warranted a family meeting. Now I was sure my appearance embarrassed them. Suddenly it seemed I had no idea what I really looked like to other people, and perhaps it was much worse than I had ever imagined. Boys would tease me about my hair until I despised them. Then the same jerks would call me at home and ask me out.

I was depressed, and there seemed to be no end in sight. School was getting harder, social rules were changing, cliques had developed, and priorities shifted to fashion and parties. I couldn't keep up. Girls and boys were commingling in a way I wasn't comfortable with. I thought most boys were morons. Suddenly everything was about how you looked and what you said.

It's funny that the things that made me an outsider back then are exactly what I like about myself today. I listened to unpopular music, wore unfashionable clothes, and didn't go to dances or parties. I developed distaste for most popular things. My attitude was caustic: "Of course you like shopping at the Limited because you're an idiot."

While I wanted to be unique, I still had a burning desire to belong, to be validated by my peers. Nothing would shut off the rotten self-talk. Most of all

I hated being me, hearing my own thoughts, having no way to remove myself from myself. I used to think, "It's not fair. I don't want to be around myself anymore than anyone else does."

At first I tried to overdose on ibuprofen, but that proved much harder than I thought. I took about twenty of them, went to sleep, and woke up in a few hours dehydrated and hungry. I went into the kitchen and ate all the leftover fried fish. That was all. Maybe being so young helped my body to bounce back.

Weeks later, I took over thirty aspirin. I lost count in the process. I don't know how many milligrams. I can't remember if I wrote a note, but it seems like my style. I put on *Sgt. Pepper's Lonely Hearts Club Band* and got into bed expecting to never wake up again. In the middle of the night, I woke up and vomited. There was nothing in my stomach anymore, but I still threw up what looked like black spit, perhaps blood. It happened several times in an hour. By the time seven o'clock rolled around, Mom told me to stay home from school. She gave me a bucket, and I lay down on the couch in the living room.

My skin was white as a sheet, and there were gray pockets beneath my eyes. Mom wasn't worried about the black vomit. She told me that was something that happened to her when she was young and drank too much alcohol. I wonder if she thought I was hung over. I didn't say anything else about it for fear that I would end up telling her the truth.

Alone, I counted the minutes between vomiting into the bucket. At first it was every eight minutes. Then every seventeen. Then every thirty-nine. So exhausted, I would fall asleep in between purging. Finally I went to sleep and didn't wake up for hours. It was over. My body recovered.

The feeling that comes from failing at suicide is different depending on whether someone knows you attempted it or not. It was just between me and myself. No one knew what was happening, and without outside interference, I just rescheduled the event. It was easy. What was frustrating was finding the most reliable method. Dying became a goal or rather a place that I just couldn't quite reach. Sadness lived in my shadow. It was the most reliable and loyal thing I'd ever known. One day, death would scoop me up in its arms and take me away from the pain. I read William Styron and began calling my self-diagnosed depression melancholia.

We had a gun, an old .45 caliber pistol. It was probably inherited from a deceased relative. Who knew how old it was or if it even worked. It was in a cabinet in the garage. I took it and put it under my bed. At first I felt relieved to have it there. To hold it in my hand was to have the definitive answer, the solution to everything. And then the reality of using it spoiled everything. Who would find me? What would be left of my face? It was more of a state-ment than I was willing to make. In the moment, the act of shooting myself seemed too real, much more real than it had in my imagination, much more difficult. I started to realize I wasn't decidedly suicidal; death wasn't the real goal. It was something else. What I really wanted was help.

During my graduate study in psychology, I would learn that this was called a "suicidal gesture" or parasuicide.[1] A person who has had many sui-cide attempts is parasuicidal. They take too many pills, but not enough to be lethal. They cut their wrists, but not deeply. They call out for help or situate themselves so they'll be found quickly. While they choose nonfatal methods, their actions are indicative of a high level of self-destructiveness. Parasuicide is most common among adolescents and young adults, and it's the strongest indicator of successful suicide in the future.

I wanted to see a psychologist, but I knew my parents wouldn't like the idea. Mom had no reaction when I told her that I needed a therapist. She seemed entirely unable to process the information. It was as if I told her something delusional. She told me to speak to my father. Dad was stunned. He thought I was being melodramatic. He told my mom to find me volunteer work. I needed to "see what a hard life is really like."

If he was trying to scare me, it must have worked. I didn't make any more attempts, although I still had thoughts. Mom never looked up volunteer work for me. Things went back to normal.

When I told Pat that I was depressed, he said, "I get down sometimes, too." I didn't tell him about the aspirin or the gun. He spent a lot more time with me in the following weeks trying to cheer me up with jokes and raunchy com-edy films. He was always good at helping me take my mind off something.

I took away several impressions from speaking to our parents about my depression, both good and bad. I thought they must be staunchly antitherapy. I felt embarrassed that I had revealed such deeply held feelings and elicited probably the worst reaction possible. Lastly, I knew I was going to have to work harder on my feelings, stop being helpless, and start fighting back. That was the lesson: the lion's share of the work was mine alone. I would go through a plethora of unhealthy ways of dealing with my depression before it finally became a thing of the past.

Entering high school, Pat wore black and listened to metal music. He wore concert T-shirts, read H. P. Lovecraft, and let his hair grow shaggy. He wanted to paint his fingernails black, but our parents wouldn't allow it. Sometimes it seemed as though he even liked being around me more than he did his friends. He listened to some of the same music as me and stopped making fun of my poetry. He learned to play "Eleanor Rigby" on the guitar, and he let me sing over it in the recording.

We'd play around with our Dad's old video camera and interview one another. "Would you rather be president or king?" I asked him.

"What kind of king? A king who has a lot of work to do or a king who's just a figurehead?"

"What difference does it make?"

"I don't want to be king just for the power," he said.

It made me feel smart to have these conversations with him, like I was mature beyond my years.

Pat was growing up to be different than most boys I knew in southeast Louisiana. He wasn't interested in duck hunting or fishing. He didn't constantly talk about the girls he met. He was, in a word, *sensitive*. He was also a cynic. Together we questioned and picked apart anything. There was a certain comfort in questioning things. When you're young, things are rather black and white. Many of the things you hold to be true are just things other people told you, not your own experience or perception. The rules at school or at home tell you what is right or wrong. Pat and I were finally realizing there was a gray area, and we loved to go looking for it. For instance, there is a fine line between being hostile and standing up for oneself. It all depends on the context. We liked to talk about things like that.

I missed seeing him at school and threw myself into a lot of new activities to make up for it. I started swimming in seventh grade, a much-needed distraction as high school approached and the world seemed to be going to bits. Pat was gone and things were changing. People were talking about where they would go to high school (a large number of children in New Orleans go to private rather than public schools). I didn't know what was happening anymore. Between kids starting to have sex, smoking weed, and taking classes based on what they would study in college, I was lost. I felt adrift in the ocean. How was I supposed to know what I wanted for my future? Every day I ordered lunch from a list of ten things they served in the cafeteria. I wasn't used to infinite possibilities.

I wasn't a great swimmer, but I loved the water. We had a wonderful team, so even being fifth place meant I was almost keeping up with some of the best swimmers in my district. My swim coach, Cameron Holt, taught me to swim when I was in first grade. He taught Pat to swim as well. Coach Cam took great pains to make the swimming pool spotless at 6:00 a.m., before we showed up for practice. When Dad had a pool put in at our house, I was mildly enthusiastic when I was asked to clean it. "Polishing my instrument," Coach called it.

Coach Cam taught children to swim in school and at camp for over twenty years. Like me, he was a fish at heart. The water made him comfortable. Just the sound of it meant that life was puttering along, leaving a playful wake, just as it should. Since he taught me to swim at age six, I had no reservations about joining the team and listening to him shout from the deck. He had a raspy voice, and you could often hear him shouting from across the lawn and through classroom windows. His glasses would slip down his sharp nose, and spittle would cling to the corner of his mouth. Kids who didn't know him were intimidated by this behavior. In fact, much of the team was also intimidated. But I wasn't. I knew him. I had known him for most of my life. I knew how to make him crack a smile, no matter how serious he could be about sports. He coached my intramural soccer team. He also taught me Louisiana history. He always shouted, but it wasn't because he was angry. He just wanted to be heard. "Smith, why are you doing that? I can't believe my eyes! How can you be doing exactly what I asked you not to do? How does that happen?" He leaned over the edge of the pool, his hands on his skinny knees. "Say it isn't so, Smith! Say it isn't so!" If anything, he was a comedian, and we were his audience.

I remember sitting out a meet against one of the strongest swim teams in our district. All of our best swimmers were going to compete. These were kids who had swum competitively since they were babies, and I knew I didn't belong to that class. I decided not to swim. I went along, carried gear, and kept time. Pat was always the captain of the tennis team or captain of the basketball team. He was the MVP, never picked last at anything he played.

Afterward we went to McDonald's, and I helped Coach rearrange equipment that had haphazardly been thrown into the back of the bus. The team was inside eating. "You eat?" he asked.

"Yeah," I lied and kept taking the boxes as he handed them to me.

"We could have used you tonight." He studied my face as he handed me another box.

"Well, this is helpful, right?" I was afraid of what he might say next.

"I like the support, I really do. But I'd like to see you get back on the horse."

"I'm going to swim next week."

"I want you to swim every week."

Someone came outside to ask him a question, and I was thankful for the respite. "Look," he resumed after the other kid went away, "I want you to keep trying. Just because you came into this later in the game than some of the other swimmers doesn't mean you can't do just as good as them. Okay?"

"Okay."

"Trust me. I know."

The way he studied my face felt like I was being dug into. I didn't want to disappoint him. I wanted to swim better. But I didn't want him to see right through me. It was obvious he did. He saw a girl that pushed herself too hard, judged herself too harshly, and retreated like a scared animal in the face of adversity. He knew I would beat myself up. He didn't let me retreat into myself and hide away. Coach didn't think I was support staff. I was the main event. I can still hear him rasp my name: "Rae, are you making mirth?"

I left co-ed school and went to a same-sex Catholic high school like Pat's. I was used to certain things like uniforms, getting demerits for eating in the classroom, and not being allowed to untuck my shirttail. What I wasn't used to was praying before every class. I had these politically incorrect religion classes where we discussed the rhythm method of family planning and the ethics of homosexual feelings. It was okay to be a homosexual, but it was a sin to act on those feelings in any way. The church also claimed that there was a time of the month when we could have sex without getting pregnant, which is important because the only purpose of sex was supposed to be procreation. We didn't believe our female teachers were using this rhythm method at home. If teachers ever got divorced, they had to renegotiate their contract to teach at the school because there was a clause that they would uphold the rules of the Catholic Church.

Although I was baptized Catholic, religion had never really been a part of my life before. Going to Catholic school was beginning to make me utterly resentful. I liked my teachers, and I loved my classmates, but the rules were absurd. There was a high level of cognitive dissonance. Doing well on a religion test meant writing an essay that, to me, was a lie. There were a number of school counselors that I could talk to about it, and I even tried. But in the end, I would sit in their office tight-lipped and then just complain about having too much homework. I even wanted to divulge my undiagnosed depression, but I was too afraid they would just advise me to pray more.

When I told Pat that I hated going to school there, he would just reassure me that it would be over someday soon. After all, he was going through the same motions at his own Catholic school. At the time he was my home base for sanity.

I stayed home on Fridays and ordered pizza—always pepperoni with extra cheese. Then Pat and I would eat and attempt to watch all the movies on AFI's Top 100. It was nice to hang out with an older kid, even if he was my brother. It felt validating. Without even realizing it, my brother encouraged and restored me. I was normal. I was better than normal: I was cool.

Pat gave me a copy of Kurt Vonnegut's *Breakfast of Champions*, and I fell in love with it. Incidentally, the novel is about Dwayne Hoover, a man who owns a car dealership, undergoing his first psychotic episode. There are many coincidences like this. Never did Pat say that he related to Dwayne Hoover or understood the way he fell to pieces. In fact, the dark oddity of the story disturbed Pat much more than it did me. I was tough. I smoked cigarettes that older kids bought me. I read books about loss and despair.

When I did have the courage to tell him what was on my mind, he had a beautiful way of giving me advice that seemed so simple it had to work: Don't let other people bother you. Keep yourself busy. Who cares what other people think? It's only important what you know.

Sometimes it was just enough to know that he knew me. He knew who I truly was and thought I was all right. Being close to Pat was knowing that people can feel as deeply as I do. As I got older I even learned that people can love you for precisely that depth of feeling.

When I felt like I didn't fit into my family, I used to think, "Well, then it's every man for himself." But now there was Pat. For the first time in my life, I felt like someone understood me. That feeling has never gone away.

For just a moment Pat was an outsider with me. Eventually Pat got a much trendier, preppy look. Sun-in streaks made his hair brassy, and he wore Tommy Hilfiger cologne. He went mainstream. His clique liked to drink on the weekends. They spent spring break in Destin chasing girls and hiding open containers from cops. It was five boys and maybe a couple of stragglers all sleeping in one dinky hotel room. He had several close friends he had known his whole life, and while I thought they were immature, they were intelligent kids. Each of them graduated high school magna cum laude or summa cum laude, and one was class salutatorian.

He returned from spring break with souvenirs for me— blown-glass fish, dolphins, and starfish. I liked knowing he thought of me while he was gone. He had a vigorous social life, never missing a weekend with the guys. Before I knew it, he even had a girlfriend. She was a blond-haired, blue-eyed girl who went to a high school I had never heard of. I thought, "He's so popular he knows people at schools all over New Orleans."

What drew people to him was his self-assuredness and sense of humor. He liked people who didn't take things too seriously, who understood there were a million perspectives on any one thing. That's probably why he studied philosophy in college. He could be silly but, if the situation called for it, sublimely practical. Reliable and responsible beyond the extent of most teenagers, he was someone you felt secure to be around. He had a great laugh and a big heart.

Sometimes his dry sense of humor offended people, but I thought it was hilarious.

"What's your dog's name?" a neighbor asked.

"Saturn," Pat answered.

"Saturn? Isn't she a girl dog? You should have named her Venus."

"No. No, I shouldn't have," he would answer in his calm monotone.

We always said Pat was the person you went to if you wanted someone to be painfully honest with you. He didn't sugarcoat his opinion. It was as if he was distinctly unable to tell a white lie. He never understood the point of it. Of course anyone can see why one might lie and say, "Oh yes, your new sofa is beautiful." Frankly, you don't have to live with that ugly sofa, so what's the point in hurting the other person's feelings? Pat didn't see it this way. For him, if you were asking his opinion, you had forfeited any right to have your feelings handled delicately. He admitted that this trait led to the end of his relationship with the blue-eyed blond and the other short-lived relationships he had in college. Sometimes he criticized himself for not "putting up" with girls, for being impatient and insensitive. Other times he felt justified in his ways. "She was self-centered and always negative about everything." There was no gray area. He didn't meet a girl halfway. Either he needed to improve himself, or she needed to improve herself. Usually the burden fell on her.

Pat knew that I was prone to sadness. I couldn't hide puffy eyes from spending an afternoon crying. He knew I spent too much time sulking in the bathtub. He knew much more than he let on because he was no stranger to pressure either. He too felt he needed to be perfect. In fact, he never did anything haphazardly. Everything he took on was something meticulously executed, whether it was sports or any other hobby. When he broke his arm he could no longer play tennis. The risk of falling on the reconstructed joint was too much. The loss of using and showing that expertise must have taken its toll.

When I was down, instead of asking me directly what was going on, he assumed that if I wanted to share it I would. He didn't want to intrude. I think he valued that kind of privacy himself, not being pushed to open up. Instead he just kept the communication open. He would suggest we do something fun together, make jokes, and try to cheer me up. If you asked him, his sister was just *moody*, like all poets.

I never went to Florida, or anywhere else, on spring break. Pat had a great deal of freedom as a teenager that I did not. People often say that's because girls can get pregnant and boys can't, but that explanation never made sense to me. It makes a number of assumptions that not only fuel misogyny but also create different pay for equal work and higher unemployment for women. Restricting and sheltering a young woman is never going to make her feel precious, but it will certainly make her naive and, in my case, angry. I was handled like something fragile. Everywhere I went, my parents called ahead. Even at sixteen, I wasn't allowed to go to the movies without an adult. By the time I was a junior in high school, it was too obvious that mine weren't like other parents. Eventually, I stopped telling them the truth about where I was going and what I was doing. If I wasn't worthy of trust, why be trustworthy?

It wasn't that easy for Pat either. While he was allowed to go out more and they didn't pry into where he was going or what he was doing, he still couldn't hang out with his friends during the week. Socializing (in person) was weekend-only in our house. Of course it made it that much more important to see our friends on the weekend. If a week went by it was like you'd missed a lifetime. As usual, Pat took it in stride, but it made me anxious.

I was painfully single, without even an admirer. I was never even sure if I was allowed to date. If it was brought up, my Dad always gave a very humorless refusal, but he admits he never took it seriously. My parents swore it wasn't because they didn't trust me that they were so strict; it was because they didn't trust what someone else might do to me. For me it felt as though they didn't trust me to make the right decisions. I thought I handled very adult situations in a mature and responsible way, but my parents didn't see that. I didn't get in cars with high or drunk kids who ended up wrapping their cars around telephone poles. I wasn't having sex. I wasn't even spending money. I saved so much shopping at thrift stores, buying ninety-nine-cent shirts.

When I compared myself to the young women I was friends with, I couldn't understand why I wasn't entrusted with the same amount of responsibility. I knew girls who ran errands for their parents every day, girls who picked up their little brothers and sisters from school. Pat was given a car at sixteen as a Christmas present. Sixteen came and went for me without a vehicle of my own. On the weekend, I needed a ride in order to go anywhere. I was allowed to use a family car only to drive to and from school. Most girls were juggling several extracurricular activities to broaden their college applications. I couldn't play sports anymore because my parents wanted me to focus on homework and studying. Other activities, like drama club and yearbook committee, would require car rides to school on the weekends, which were difficult to attain. For one thing, we lived nearly forty miles away from my high school. Secondly, most people my age weren't interested in going anywhere near school at noon on Saturday.

Unlike Pat, I stayed counterculture. Soon I began to seek out things just because other people didn't like them. I started wearing very loose clothing, large threadbare T-shirts, and baggy scrub pants. I shopped in the little boys' section at department stores. I chopped my hair off, dyed it funky colors, and shunned makeup. I knew it wasn't flattering, but for me the point was to hide myself. I didn't want anyone to approach me because they liked the way my body looked. I had no interest in that kind of attention. You had to really know me in order to like me.

Without the distraction of boys and sex, I had plenty of time to work on my creative side. I took every artistic elective and found new ways to draw, decoupage, and plaster. I bought little kid toothbrushes with Cookie Monster and Big Bird on them, boiled them until they were soft and the bristles fell out, and then bent them into bangles.

My dad didn't mind my new look at all. I think he liked my green-blue hair. He thought I was bold, not the run-of-the-mill teenager. His attitude was, "Well, if she can dye it blond, then she can dye it pink or purple or whatever else she likes." I ran wild with that. Mom, on the other hand, seemed disturbed by it. Her little girl went from having her hair professionally straightened and getting manicures to cutting her own hair and carefully avoiding ever looking pretty. In her mind, there were much nicer clothes I could wear and still be modest. In Dad's mind, "We'd better get the storage boxes down from the attic. I'm sure I have some shirts and sweaters up there she'd like."

I worked hard to get comfortable in my own skin, but there was just not enough encouragement in the world to stop the negative self-talk. Although some would say I embraced the title, I didn't enjoy feeling like a freak. There was a lot more to me than my looks, and Pat might have been the only person to see that. He never put me down for the way I dressed. He probably even liked that the androgynous look his little sister adopted was keeping a lot of boys away.

Depression was still always one step behind me. I was my own worst enemy. I took in information from the world around me and skillfully managed to make all of it mean something negative about myself. Everything was my fault. I felt bad because I deserved to feel bad. I'd stop writing or painting and want to tear it up, ruin the canvas, or throw it away. In the back of my mind, the voice would resound, "You'll never get away no matter how hard you try"—self-hate so thick I could swim in it. I finally decided to do something about it other than suicide.

I broke a compact mirror and used the pieces to cut my arm. It seemed instinctual that it would give me relief. Seeing blood and feeling the pain felt like a release. Cutting was fitting punishment, and the result was unrelenting calm like none I'd ever felt before. It almost put me to sleep. I didn't want drugs or alcohol. I believed self-harm was a perfectly viable way of managing my feelings, and I was proud of myself for having found such a good solution.

Sometimes I hid my cuts well, but the ones done in a moment of impulse could be anywhere. I liked to punch things. Bloody knuckles were quick to accomplish and extremely relieving. Of course, hands are hard to hide, especially in the summertime. I remember Pat asking me about the marks on my fist. I told him I was angry and punched something. It was clear he related; a lot of guys feel pent-up aggression in adolescence. But he had never done something that reckless to himself. He tried to make light of it, the way he did with most things: "Maybe next time you can punch one of the twenty pillows you have on your bed."

I couldn't say, "No, there has to be pain and blood." Cutting was my biggest secret. Other things were obvious: suicide was a desire to die, depression was chronic unhappiness, and drug use was an escape. But self-harm was harder to explain. I didn't know anyone else who did it. I had no idea that other people even did it at all, let alone that they got the same immense satisfaction it gave me. I believed it was truly freakish. But Pat never treated me that way. In Pat's eyes, I was just his sister. I was never an unsolvable problem or an outsider.

Part 2

COMING APART

6

Turbulent Teens

While we were in high school, our parents began spending less time together. Dad would stay late at the office and come home to a ten o'clock dinner. Half asleep, Mom would still be waiting to eat. Despite the fact that he was usually late, she'd still wait for him, almost defiantly. They often fell asleep in the living room on separate couches. The fact that they were drifting apart was unspoken. There weren't any fights. Sometimes there was tension beneath the surface. It didn't seem like we as a family were falling apart, because their relationships with Pat and me got stronger during this time. Each of them went out of their way to spend more one-on-one time with us. Initially I found it intrusive, but then I realized they just wanted to be with us. It was a nice feeling.

Mom spent more time with Pat. He was always closer to her. In family discussions, they were always a sounding board for each other. I spent more time with Dad because we had similar interests. Sometimes we would get up early in the morning to go fishing. We watched horror films, old episodes of *Alfred Hitchcock Presents*, and racy cartoons like *South Park*. He took me to Arkansas one weekend to pick up my grandmother, and on the way there I read Richard Matheson's *I Am Legend* to him in its entirety. "He's the last man on earth and the rest are all vampires?" He was on the edge of his seat.

Mom and I didn't like the same things. I thought the shows she watched were stupid, and she thought the places I shopped were gross. Most of my girlfriends didn't have close relationships with their mothers. It was almost a rite of passage to reject them during adolescence. It wasn't so bad at first, but then our relationship turned toxic. She grew increasingly strict, insisting she was worried about me, about the young woman I was becoming. I thought that she just didn't like my baggy clothes and wild hair colors, but she explained to me later on in life that she began focusing on me instead of the problems that arose in her marriage. She said she thought that doing this would get my dad more involved, more engaged as a husband. Instead, Dad seemed to think she was being critical of him as a parent.

Suddenly she wanted to know every last detail of my social activities. Several times I found her outside my bedroom eavesdropping while I used the phone. When I asked Pat what I should do, he said, "Just don't lie to her. It obviously makes her mad."

"But I have to lie. Otherwise she won't let me do anything. I can't even go to the movies without a parent."

He shrugged. "Then don't get caught in the lie."

"It's not fair. You never had to follow rules like that. You've never even had a curfew."

"That's because I can't get pregnant," he smirked. Throughout his teens, when he went out, no one even asked him where he was going or who he was with. He had never been grounded. His nights out usually included underage drinking. He came home once with a mysterious abrasion across his chin and cheek. He later told me it was from blacking out and hitting his face on the pavement in the French Quarter. Now he was a senior in high school, and he came and went as he pleased. Considering new developments with Mom, I didn't think I'd ever get to that point.

I didn't think it was fair. As a sophomore in high school, all I understood was that the window of freedom I once had was getting smaller. Meanwhile girls around me were getting their driver's licenses. I couldn't accept rides from other teens, except for Pat. I couldn't date. If I went to a friend's house and their parents were not home, I was to go home immediately. If there were boys around, I definitely had to get home. I looked for ways to keep busy, even trying out for the cross-country team at school. Then I found out I wasn't allowed to participate in team sports because it would take time away from my studies.

It was very difficult to get my friends to cooperate with all these conditions because they didn't have any rules like that. Mom would call their parents to get details about my visits. The other parents were confused, if not wary. They treated me differently after that. I imagine they thought I was doing drugs or stealing things, something significant that made my mom suddenly so concerned.

If she caught me in a lie, even if I just failed to disclose every name from a gathering I attended, it would require a serious discussion. She would tell Dad, "We need to talk about Sarah." She never grounded me herself, always leaving the punishment up to Dad, but she would let him know it if she thought he was too lenient.

Eventually, he didn't even want to have the discussion. "What do you want me to say?" he'd sigh. "Just tell her she's grounded yourself."

Getting grounded was Draconian in our household. It lasted for an indeterminate amount of time and encompassed any activity outside of the home. I was only allowed to go to school and places with Mom. Nothing else. I had no idea when the arrangement would end. I was bored and restless, isolated. Pat was rarely home, and my friends didn't want to come over because they feared that my parents were so strict they wouldn't approve of them. My relationship with Dad deteriorated. When he would be friendly and kind, I resented the fact that I was still perpetually grounded. Most of our conversations became arguments, until we rarely spoke at all.

Pat stayed out of it, probably happy not to be in trouble himself. I think I would have done the same if the tables were turned. The most baffling thing about it was that it came down to brass tacks. I was a good kid. No one would have argued otherwise, except Mom. It hurt me that she imagined I was on the road to ruin, despite the many times I had weathered troubled waters to avoid just that. So many kids from school were doing drugs like ketamine and crystal meth, and some even began selling them. I quickly distanced myself from them. At sixteen, a good friend of mine became pregnant. She kept the baby. I wasn't even sexually active.

But there didn't seem to be any point in playing it safe. Mom's watchful eye made me feel like a criminal. Good behavior wasn't cutting me any breaks, so I started sneaking out of my window at night to find whatever kind of trouble I could get into. I made a number of new counterculture friends who took me to raves and punk shows. Most of them were straightedge. They didn't use drugs, not even caffeine. I was the vegan of the group, swearing off a wide array of things just because it felt good to be in control. But I did find myself curious about mood-altering drugs. I skipped marijuana and went straight to ecstasy. It was easy to get one's hands on X at raves, even if it was twenty-five dollars a pill. I remember feeling exhilarated. I couldn't find a thing in the world that made me unhappy while I was rolling. But it was an all-night drug. I was high until I went to bed. When I woke up in the morning I was sore in places I never knew I had. It wasn't for me. The kind of happiness I felt on X was something I was pretty sure I could simulate without the drug. I thought of it as a model for beating depression and battling self-consciousness.

There was a person I was sure I wanted to be. It's hard to remember now, but I wished to be more spontaneous. I wanted to be able to let things roll off my back. Stop being so serious. Stop feeling like every decision I made or action I took carried the weight of the world. I had been taught that there was but one right way to do anything, and you either did it that way or you failed. A misstep wasn't something that could be corrected. If you lost a foothold, there was no net. It made me an anxious person. All the while something inside me yearned to throw it down and run free. If only I didn't feel so certain that things wouldn't work out. Pat felt the pressure too. We worried we'd never be able to stand on our own two feet. We felt like overgrown children. Security was tenuous and fleeting. Adulthood was upon us, and it didn't feel like we had earned it at all.

When Pat graduated high school and went to college, a part of me went up in flames. I was grounded so often that in a week he might be the only friend I got to speak to. I wasn't ready to come home from school to an empty house. With Pat gone and Dad not coming home until late, it would just be Mom and me all night. Dinner was silent and strained.

I kept finding myself going to his bedroom door, and just before knocking I'd remember he wasn't there. I didn't know who to talk to about school, friends, or family. I felt socially awkward and wanted his advice: Did I do something weird? Is it normal to feel this way? I wanted reassurance.

Every family get-together was unbearable without him. I still have dreams where my whole family is over, and Pat and I are sitting together talking and laughing. Together we are our own little island, where the weather is calm, where the locals are sincerely friendly and life is simple.

One night Mom found me napping in Pat's bed. I told her that him going off to college felt like the end of something, like we had crossed over a point and could never return. She said she was happy that I grasped the fact that we were "growing up." She said a lot of people pass over that moment and only miss it in retrospect. I felt like she didn't really understand what I meant. I wanted to shake her and say, "Don't you see? He's the only good thing about this family."

I could get through the day at school just fine. But as 3:30 rolled around, I dreaded going home. It made me feel so empty. I took solace in our dogs. Pat always took such great care of them that I was determined to keep that up. I even let the oldest dog sleep in my bed at night, no matter how smelly or restless she became.

Pat came home nearly every weekend. He said he felt obligated; "guilty" was the word he used. I don't know if he felt he had to see our parents or if he had to see me. It cheered me up nonetheless. I had so much to tell him by the end of the week. We'd go outside late at night to sneak cigarettes, and I'd sit on top of the gray, plastic garbage can telling him about this and that. He was usually in good spirits, but I knew he resented never getting to do things with his college friends on the weekend. He missed out on a lot, and the ties loosened. He never regained that closeness he once had with the guys.

He didn't make many new friends in college. He spent most of his time in his apartment smoking marijuana. His friends would have to go over to his place if they wanted to see him. He didn't like to go out and wasn't interested in parties. He spent most of his cash on video games and weed. He smoked every day and mentioned to me that it had tripped up his schedule at school a few times. He missed classes he didn't mean to miss, one day skipping an exam. He met with the professor and was honest with him: "I just screwed up. I have no excuse." Taken aback with Pat's honesty, the teacher was appreciative and let him make up the test.

Weed was his new best friend. He'd bring it home with him on the weekend, and we would smoke together at night. I never got the satisfaction from it that he did. It just made me sleepy. When Pat talked about the way marijuana made him feel, it was like he was talking about a miracle drug. He knew how to rig anything into a pipe. He had numerous places to stash weed. When he ran out, he'd scrape the bowl meticulously with a paper clip, roll the black resin into a ball, and smoke that. I marveled at how much he had picked up, but I wasn't worried about him. Marijuana seemed really harmless, especially when compared to the cigarettes we smoked. But it was his avid dedication to getting high that frightened me. It was something that had to be done, smoking over and over. It was so important that I began to wonder who was in control: the person or the craving. Was it a desire or a compulsion? Smoking weed was the goal of the day. It was the reward that Pat worked toward. He always had some on him. There were worse drugs he could have been using. He had tried ecstasy and peyote but said they weren't really for him. Rather than grow concerned or scared, I just thought, "Well, he's in college. This is what college kids do."

One day he did open up to me about his new habit. Apparently he was having social anxiety, and marijuana helped him to feel more natural and laid back. "I just feel so uncomfortable in groups of people, around strangers. It's just *unease*."

"I understand what you mean." The news floored me. I had no idea Pat had those feelings too. "That's why I don't like parties."

"I feel like everyone's watching me."

"And judging."

"Like I look like an idiot."

"I know exactly how you feel. It's like I can't be myself. I get clumsy."

"I don't know if I get clumsy, but I don't feel happy. If I don't like socializing, then why should I do it?"

"Because people think that being extroverted is right. Being shy is bad and wrong. It's a flaw."

"Is that what it is? Introversion?"

I nodded. "Some people like to be with people, and other people prefer to be alone."

We looked up "introversion" on the Internet and found a bunch of sites on how to overcome it. Pat was interested in reading them to make himself feel more comfortable in groups, but I thought the how-to lists were insulting. When we searched for "extroversion," there were no websites on how to "overcome" it. We did learn that extroverts are considered to be people who derive energy from being with others, whereas introverts are energized by having time to themselves. We were satisfied with that. We could acknowledge the discomfort of socializing without feeling guilty anymore.

Talking to a lot of people often made me feel tired. If someone slept over on Friday night, I was ready for them to go home Saturday morning. My Mom related. She called it needing "time to unwind and decompress." For as long as I can remember I never liked going to parties, but I wasn't necessarily aware of any feelings of anxiety. I just didn't think of a party as a fun place to be. I'd rather go to the movies or just have dinner with a couple of friends. Introversion didn't hold me back or keep me from doing the things I wanted, but social anxiety did. Having to go to new places alone would cause great distress for me, but I never understood why. I would have trouble focusing on anything else for a week, maybe even a month beforehand. I don't know what I thought the worst thing was that could happen. Looking stupid? Lost? Being observed by a great number of people at once? Even giving book reports to a classroom of students I had known my whole life was insurmountable. I thought about having to give the report every day I walked into the classroom, all semester, until I had done the presentation.

The thing I didn't realize back then was that Pat didn't have the same pattern as me. Growing up, he had been a social butterfly. He often led the group, was the center of attention, and never seemed ill at ease. When he disclosed his social anxiety to me, he wasn't telling me an old secret. He was telling me about something new, an anxiety that had only recently cropped up. It was specific to being around people, especially strangers.

Pat often gave me rides around town. Even if I was grounded, I was allowed to go anywhere with my brother. He'd take me to my friend's house and pick me up the next day. Sometimes we'd slip in an impromptu movie. It was exhilarating for me because I never got to do anything else without getting permission from our parents. But not when I was with Pat. We'd go get coffee and sneak cigarettes. We perfumed ourselves on the way home. I can still remember the smell of his old Civic: smoke covered up by "new car" air freshener.

One weekend stands out to me now. Pat was nineteen and I was seventeen. A new Wes Anderson movie called *The Royal Tenenbaums* had just opened. Pat had chosen the film; frankly I knew nothing about it. We bought tickets at the box office and proceeded upstairs to the theater. But once we got there we saw a roped-off queue to get in. "It's opening weekend," I explained to him.

He gave one of those gruff sighs that told me he was overwhelmed. There were only about five people in line, and our odds were still good at getting a nice seat. But he said, "Look, can we just go? I'll make it up to you if we can just go home. Here," he handed me some cash to pay me back for my ticket. He promised again, "I'll make it up to you."

I shrugged my shoulders, and we went home. Pat didn't like lines. He didn't like waiting. At the time I thought, "He's just the type of guy who likes to get in and out of a place fast." He didn't go to a store without knowing what he wanted first. He could get in and out of a shopping mall in ten minutes flat. But there was more to it than that. I didn't realize at the time that he hadn't always been that way. He didn't always get flustered in public. When we were little, he was never overwhelmed by a crowd.

The onset of Pat's schizophrenia is considered insidious rather than acute. His symptoms didn't flood in all at once. His symptoms started small and grew into more significant, glaring problems. By early adulthood, he had changed from an extroverted person with little anxiety to an introverted person who disliked crowds, avoided most social events, and felt social anxiety. Changes came so gradually that he always just seemed like the same old Pat. Years later when a psychiatrist would ask us about this, he was alarmed. He told us that a change in disposition like that is highly unusual.

I'm sure there were many changes that we never noticed, little things that were insignificant. But I wonder now, if Pat hadn't become a more anxious and withdrawn person like me, would we have been so close to begin with? I can't be sure. All I know is that the following Christmas, Pat gave me a DVD: *The Royal Tenenbaums*.

Grounded most weekends and feeling that I'd lost my place in the world now that Pat had moved out, right on time a girl walked into my life. She wasn't even a girl. She was a woman: twenty years old, while I was only sixteen. She was a friend of a friend. For some reason, she saw me as an equal, a kindred spirit. With short blue hair, tattoos, and multiple piercings, her attention was always on me no matter how many others were around. We started spending a lot of time together. I finally confronted feelings that had plagued me for years, urges that made going to an all-girls school very difficult. I was in love. She wasn't the first girl I'd had feelings for, but it was the first time the relationship was out in the open. Outright, with nothing to hide, Mira was my girlfriend.

Other girls had been secretive. They weren't usually from my circle of friends. One girl would slip notes in my locker, obscure poetry hinting at mutual attraction. In the end I slept over at her house one night. For the most part, after a sexual encounter, these young women would retreat into their old lives like it had never happened. They had sought me out probably because of my short hair and androgynous clothes, thinking I might help them explore their bisexual fantasies. Like ships passing in the night, some acted like it was nothing, like it was just an accident, a momentary lapse of heterosexuality. I don't know if they felt guilt, shame, or just an inability to face the truth. I was left to feel like I had taken advantage of *them* somehow. There was no intimacy between us. They wanted to forget anything had happened between us.

Mira embraced our relationship. She was proud to introduce me to her friends and family. But seeing Mira was complicated. I had to sneak around at all hours of the night. My parents didn't want me anywhere near her. They said she was too old to be hanging around sixteen-year-olds. Of course, that made no sense to me then. Once I was nineteen years old and we had broken up, I couldn't possibly imagine hanging around anyone in high school, let alone dating a sixteen-year-old.

When I told Pat I was seeing a girl, he was shocked but not judgmental. He had a lot of questions and didn't want to hurt my feelings. "So, are you a lesbian now?"

"I guess so," was my answer. It was very confusing because I didn't feel I could say I was bisexual because I had never been with a man, and yet I was attracted to men. I had kissed a boy once at a rave, but I never called him again. So I told Pat I was gay, and he asked for permission to talk to his best friend Tom about it. I thought that was cute. I told him of course, he had every right to want to talk to his best friend about it.

A lot of our friends said they thought it was very predictable, and yet it was always a mystery to me. I didn't know how I felt about men or women; I just knew I couldn't help what sex I was attracted to. Sex was a nonissue. It was about the person and how well we connected. When I explained all of this to Pat, he wasn't put off at all. Rather he was intrigued. "How long did you know you liked girls?"

I thought back as far as I could. "I guess I always did."

"I always did too," he snickered. I felt as though he accepted me just the way I was. We agreed not to tell my parents. We both had secrets to keep.

Then I got caught skipping school to see Mira, and I was grounded for over a year. Spending all my free time sneaking around with her, I began to lose touch with my friends. By the time I finished high school, I hardly knew what was going on in their lives.

The day after I graduated, I packed a car with my things. I drove to New Orleans and dropped off my stuff at Mira's house. I took the car to my grandmother's house and put all the keys in her mailbox. I called my mother and told her where to find the keys. I said, "I'm leaving."

She said, "Oh no you're not!"

I hung up the mobile phone and put that in the mailbox too. Those last words frightened me. When I think of it now, I still feel a cold chill on my back. I spent a week looking over my shoulder. Every time Mira and I stopped at a red light, my heart would lurch and I'd imagine someone would open my door and pull me from the car. I thought the police were looking for me. I wondered if I had been reported missing. Mira was carefree. She wanted to do all the things we never got to do before like go to the movies, the beach, and parties. She wanted me to get that nose ring I always wanted and get matching tattoos. There were people she wanted me to finally meet, but none of them seemed to grasp the gravity of the situation. No one knew that I had left home, that my parents were likely distraught, and that they might not want to speak to me again. All I wanted to do was cry. I was too afraid to go anywhere for nine days. On the ninth day, I called Pat.

"Hello? Pat, it's me. It's Sarah."

"Sarah?" his voice cracked. "Wait, wait a minute. I'm at school." I heard him rushing about. He got back into his car, where he could speak privately. He was bawling. "Sarah, where are you? What happened?" I had never seen or heard my brother cry before.

"Everything is okay. I'm in New Orleans with Mira. I moved in with her."

"Nobody knew where you were! It's—it's like you're dead."

"I'm fine. Everything's fine." I was shocked.

"They're holding a meeting at the house today. The whole family is there. Mom and Dad are telling everyone you've run away."

"I didn't run away. I'm eighteen and a half. I just moved out."

"Sarah, you just disappeared."

"I'm not far away. You can always reach me."

"I can see you?"

"Of course you can!"

"Tomorrow? Can I see you tomorrow?"

"Sure, of course. We'll get coffee. You can finally meet Mira."

He sniffled and sounded a little calmer. "Okay. Okay, that sounds good."

His emotional outburst broke my heart. How could he think anything would ever keep me from him? I had told him a year earlier about my plans to leave home, but I don't think he believed me. He probably just thought I was blowing off steam for being grounded. I was careful not to remind him of it, in case he tried to stop me. The fact that he missed me and wasn't angry helped me to relax a little. He was the first thread I could tie together between my old life and my new one. Now, if I could only get our folks on board.

7

Arrest and the First Psychologist

My girlfriend Mira didn't understand all my stress and sleeplessness when I moved in with her. She was unable to empathize and see my position. I remember telling her, "I've sacrificed so much."

Then she asked, "What? What did you sacrifice?"

After nine months, I moved out of her house. Living together had been a real eye-opener. She didn't work or go to school. She slept until four in the afternoon, spent all night in bars, and returned home around sunrise. She was immature, which may explain why she was seeking the company of teenagers.

Something incredible did come from our short-lived relationship. It was the first time I had made a misstep and didn't beat myself up about it. Instead of retreating into a dark place and rubbing my nose in my mistakes, I believed I had done my best. My friends and even some of Mira's were very supportive of the split. Some never understood what I was doing with a much older person, especially since I was often supporting her financially. I was hopeful, and although things didn't work out, I felt like I matured out of that relationship. I was in contact with my parents, but we rarely spoke. I moved in with Maw-Maw Alice, and she seemed to enjoy my company.

During the summer of 2003, Pat went on a tubing trip upstate with some old friends. Because a lot of underage drinking goes on in the waterways, police set up checkpoints in the woods. They watch for illicit behavior from the high banks, shielded by the tree line, and stop tubers as they come downriver. They caught Pat and several of his friends smoking marijuana from a pipe. The boys dumped most of it into the water immediately. The police estimated it wasn't much, and they asked whose it was. The boys, then twenty years old, looked at each other. Pat instinctively said, "It was mine. The pipe is mine too."

Although all the boys were smoking, only Pat was taken to the police station and booked. He was charged with a misdemeanor possession, which entailed a fine, and our parents were called to pick him up. Because of his self-effacing demeanor and politeness, officers agreed not to put him in lockup and instead let him stay seated at the booking officer's desk.

I don't know how much of the weed or the paraphernalia actually belonged to Pat, but I know the boys with him also purchased and smoked weed on a daily basis. He described the incident by saying, "I decided I'd take the fall." The police said as much to our parents. Mom and Dad were bewildered, embarrassed, and disappointed. Mom was upset that he took the blame, and it changed the way she viewed Pat's friends. Dad could hardly speak or even look at him.

It's hard to tell looking back if your parents were negligent for not realizing you were into something bad right under their noses or if you were just that clever when it came to sneaking around. I think any parent would like to believe that their kid wasn't smoking marijuana, no matter how innocuous they might consider the drug, because it is an illegal substance. No responsible parent can get behind an illegal substance.

They asked Pat, "Why? How could you do this? You have everything. We give you everything." He finally spilled the beans about his social anxiety. When he told me this, I was surprised they took it seriously. "They didn't think that was a real explanation, right? You smoke weed even when you're alone."

"I wouldn't smoke as much if it weren't for the anxiety."

That's when I knew Pat wasn't like other college students. This habit wasn't a phase. It wasn't a momentary escape or an experiment. It was self-medication.

"They want me to see a psychologist," he said.

"They what?" I was flabbergasted.

"They want me to get help for my social anxiety. I have an appointment with a psychologist on Wednesday."

"Which one suggested the doctor? Mom or Dad?"

"I don't know. Both of them, I guess."

"You're kidding."

"Not at all."

"Don't you think that's weird? I always thought they hated psychologists, especially Dad."

"I never got that impression."

"Don't you remember what he told me when I was twelve and suicidal?"

"No. What are you talking about?"

"Never mind."

"I'm leaving Baton Rouge and moving back to New Orleans. I'm enrolling at UNO."

"Really?" I could barely hide my excitement. I was attending the University of New Orleans, and I was happy to have my brother at school with me for the first time since we were kids.

"Yeah, it's a good idea. I wasn't doing well in the business program, and I want to change majors. I'm thinking philosophy."

"Wow, so this is a big life change for you." Pat majored in business, and I never understood why. It was like he didn't have a choice. It was just the most logical step to take. When he took philosophy as an elective, he seemed to get much more out of it.

"It'll be good. I just wasn't that happy in Baton Rouge."

"Well, I'd be happy to show you around."

Pat wasn't interested in meeting many of my friends at school. I did notice once or twice that we'd be crossing campus, and he'd run into an old buddy from high school. They would stop and chat for a second, but Pat always looked like he was in a hurry to get away, even when he had nowhere else to be. He'd hustle along as if he wasn't interested in friendships, old or new. He was all business. You couldn't find him cutting up and smoking cigarettes with other kids on the quad. He didn't go to the cafeteria, the library, or the lounge. We got lunch together off campus, but usually if he wasn't in class he went to work. Because it was a family business, Dad hired us as clerks and let us work odd hours around our course schedules. Pat wasn't just standoffish; he seemed to be stuck up. He wasn't interested in meeting any new people, but he hadn't been that way before. I told myself that maybe he just didn't like many people.

A year after moving out of the family home, I began to recover my relationship with my parents. Dad offered me a job at his office working side by side with Pat. Much of that was facilitated by my brother. He had long talks with Dad about me and helped him open up a little and let me back into his life. I think he feared getting hurt again. Mom, surprisingly, was the one quick to forgive me. She embraced seeing me every day and seemed genuinely happy to have me back.

My extended family hadn't been surprised about me dating a girl. At twenty-one, I shared a cigarette with my Aunt Sue. She said, "They told me you were seeing that girl, and I was like, 'Okay. What else is new?'" she laughed. It was comforting to laugh about it, and nice to hear that not only did she see it coming, but it wasn't a big deal to her. My next serious relationship with a big, burly guy didn't shock or amaze anyone either. I was an unusual girl with eclectic taste, and no one expected to predict my next move.

My relationship with Mira may be the only thing I ever look back on and wish I could change. The entire experience sent my anxiety into a tailspin. Meeting her and determining that I wanted to move out made me think, "I have to be more serious, more responsible, more grown up." That translated into planning everything, worrying more and more. I would plan most things in advance to a tee, and then ruminate on any way in which it didn't go exactly as planned. My mind was always in the future, and I often missed out on the here and now. But for some reason I thought this was the key to being responsible. Always waiting for the other shoe to drop, I moved from one worry to the next. I would zoom in so tightly on the things that were imperfect in life, the things that needed the most work, that I missed all the sweetness in life.

This is something I have spent my whole life working to undo. There are places I want to go and people I want to meet, but it's exhausting fighting my fear of the unknown. There are so many things I have missed because I was too afraid to do it on my own. As I approach thirty, I still have so much work to do. Before I go to a social event, I have to avoid thinking about the possible scrutiny I might undergo there; otherwise I might back out. There are many times I find myself about to worry excessively over something in the future, and I have to pause and tell myself, "Life is big. Life is much bigger than this one thing you're about to worry sick over."

Pat's attitude of seeming above everyone, above socializing, appealed to me back then. It's one of the ways we grew together more closely when he began his descent into schizophrenia. While I was ashamed of being too nervous to show up at a music venue by myself, Pat would just shrug it off like it was nothing. He was the guy who'd say, "Yeah, I didn't go to my friend's wedding. So what?" It wasn't until months would pass without Pat so much as talking on the phone with one of his friends that I worried his withdrawal was more than just being elitist. Social withdrawal is a common symptom of schizophrenia. Many families report it as being one of the first changes they noticed.[1]

His psychologist, Dr. Milner, was a jovial man in his early seventies. Born and educated in the Midwest, Milner specialized in family counseling. His fingernails were always manicured, and he wore button-downs printed with crawfish and gumbo pots. Always smiling, he struck me as a man who was already retired, already on vacation.

For his anxiety, Pat was prescribed an antidepressant often used to treat panic disorder and generalized anxiety disorder. Pat found Dr. Milner very easy to talk to and had me come into some sessions with him to corroborate and help him remember certain events. After solo sessions, Pat would often come visit me. He'd smoke a cigarette and tell me about his session, how he learned something new or saw something differently afterward. He seemed to use therapy by and large as a way of "social checking." He would recount events to the doctor, how they made him feel and how he reacted, and would essentially want to know, "Is this socially right? Is it normal and okay?"

Pat was very hopeful that the medication would ease his anxiety, but less than a month into taking it he was already saying, "It's not working. I don't feel any different." I urged him to give it some more time, but eventually he stopped taking the antidepressant. He started smoking marijuana again, although less often than before. I was just happy that he was seeing Dr. Milner on a regular basis. I believed he would work out his anxiety over time in session, even if it took years. I didn't think about the fact that Pat considered his anxiety to be something out of his control. He didn't know where it came from, and he didn't feel like he could change it. It simply happened to him. While I didn't have my own anxiety under control, I did believe it was something I could learn to change. We were both experiencing something called anxiety, and yet I was the only one attributing that anxiety to thoughts and perceptions under my control. Meanwhile he felt immense fear and stress in social situations, and he could not understand where these feelings were coming from.

I can understand how those circumstances could lead to feelings of paranoia. But I don't remember him ever talking about anything paranoid before
the age of twenty-four. There was only one occasion when he said something
to me that I didn't quite believe, but he seemed utterly convinced of it. He and
I went to different high schools. I was just seventeen when I got in trouble at
my high school for truancy. The school's disciplinarian had a long talk with
me about why I had skipped school. Afterward she complimented me for being so forthcoming. I thought, well, of course. The jig is up. What else could
I say? "No, I really was at school. I was just invisible that day"?

Pat said that the reason the disciplinarian wanted to speak to me about
the incident was not because she wanted to know the truth. Rather she just
wanted to see if I'd tell her the truth. "They probably have a whole file on you.
That's what they had at my school."

"What do you mean?"

"At my high school they knew what you were up to outside of school. They
had sources."

I didn't believe him. My school disciplinarian didn't seem to know very
much about me. After all, we had never spoken before this occasion. Furthermore she didn't even ask me about my life at home. It was as if she didn't
want to know much, lest she have to do something about it. "She didn't seem
to know anything other than what I told her."

"Maybe not at your school, but mine knew everything about us."

"How do you know?"

"Other students. People told me."

He didn't say any more than that, and I didn't pry. I knew he had a friend
who was sent to rehab during high school for amphetamine abuse, and perhaps he felt like the faculty had played a role in the intervention. Despite what
he said, I thought he was giving the administration at both schools far too
much credit. Being private, I noticed they tiptoed around making waves with
our tuition-paying parents as much as possible. I don't know a single student
expelled from my high school who wasn't eventually asked to come back.

In Terry Gilliam's 1985 film *Brazil* about a future, dystopian society in
which Big Brother is always watching, there is a sign with a totalitarian government slogan that reads, "Suspicion Breeds Confidence." When I saw that
film, I remembered what Pat had said about his high school spying on students. Part of me wondered if Pat liked to imagine there was a "file" on him

out there in order to make himself feel special. He was always so reasonable, and yet in this case I couldn't make him see how silly this conspiracy theory sounded. Therefore if he bought into this crazy idea, I figured it served him in some way to believe it. If one was convinced people were always watching him, it might lead him to be a perfectionist. If you're forever observed and scrutinized, you had better be on your best behavior. Perhaps this is why Pat was such a great high school student and graduated with honors. When he went to college, his grades dipped and he rarely went to class. Had Big Brother stopped watching, or was he just tired of putting on the performance? Either way, I can see where this belief about being monitored would cause a great deal of social anxiety.

I remember when he transferred to my college like it was yesterday. Having trouble finding parking, I was a few minutes late to the first day of Modern European History class. I sat down as the professor began to call roll. When I heard my last name, I called out, "Here."

He marked it down and then he said my name again, "Rae?"

"Um," I hesitated because that had never happened before.

"Here," Pat said from several rows away. Our eyes met, and I smiled. The professor continued down the list. It's hard to explain how happy it made me that Pat was taking this elective. He hadn't told me anything about his schedule, and, being several years behind him, I never thought we'd run into each other in school. It was the first and only time I ever had a class with my brother.

History met just before lunchtime, and afterward we both had a break. We'd usually leave campus for food and rush back to make it to our next classes. Neither of us ever missed a day of that course. While Pat was working hard not to fall back into his old habits of skipping classes and smoking weed, I went to class just to see him. I never passed on lunch with him to do things with other friends. Frankly, hanging out with Pat was better than being with my own friends. We had more in common, and he knew me better than anyone. We studied together before exams. He would come over to Maw-Maw Alice's with his books, usually spending the night. Pat was still smoking marijuana, but much less than before. After we hit the books, he'd smoke marijuana and I would smoke my cigarettes. Then we watched cartoons.

That semester I struggled with an elective sociology course I was taking. It was the kind of class that's packed with a hundred freshmen and sophomores on day one. Two weeks into the semester, only a third of them remain. The ideas were just too big. The young professor, a graduate student himself, had assumed too much about his students. He thought we were in tune to world news, the IMF, apartheid, outsourcing, the Treaty on the Non-Proliferation of Nuclear Arms. He talked about abstract concepts and then tested us by asking us to parse how those concepts would play out in different contexts. These were essay examinations. He wasn't asking us to regurgitate the textbook or lecture. He wanted a critique from us. No matter how much I studied the material, I wasn't able to use it. As Pat put it, I thought too small. I needed to learn to consider more expansive factors, the macro level of social structure. When I went over the study guide with him, he was amused and excited about the material. Ever the patient tutor, he'd try to get me to open up my mind. "You know what would have helped you a lot in high school?" he asked.

"What?"

"A Model United Nations."

"We didn't have a Model UN." It sounded boring. It's highly unlikely I would have taken part in that.

"That's a shame. It could really get you thinking about stuff like this," he said, although he didn't participate in Model UN either.

He wasn't angry, disappointed, or superior when I slipped up. Instead he'd help me formulate a response to each question, hitting upon the main points I should make, trying to get me to come up with the ideas on my own. Of course, not everything on the study guide would be on the exam, but we went through it all. I know I passed that class because he helped me. His grades always confirmed he was a smart guy, but his intellect never intimidated me until I was working on something *with* him. Unlike me, he was able to keep many factors in mind at once and parse out his ideas in a way that would make sense to anyone. He wasn't just some college dummy getting high and spending his parents' money. I knew he was going to finish his degree in philosophy with a stellar GPA. I wasn't worried about the arrest or the weed.

8

Living Together: Less Marijuana, More Beer

When I moved out of my parents' house, I feared my relationship with Pat would wither away, but we still saw a lot of each other. In 2004, we even moved into a house together. Our parents bought a second home, a house that used to belong to an elderly relative. It was close to our college, and they let Pat and me move in. It was a three-bedroom, fairly new, mostly furnished, and we only had to pay utilities. The master suite belonged to our parents, although they never stayed over.

That left Pat and me to negotiate who would end up with the tiny bedroom. It was better suited to be a study or maybe a separate den. I couldn't fit both my bed and my computer desk inside it, but I took it anyway. My reasoning was that I would spend more time out of the house than Pat, so it was better for him to have the roomier accommodation. He only went to work, school, and the grocery store—just the essential places. Still there was always a part of me that expected Pat to start doing more things with me. A lot of his friends went to school elsewhere. But I had a nice group of friends, some older and some younger, and they welcomed Pat with open arms. He never wanted to go anywhere with me, though. He might ask me to bring him an iced coffee or a pack of cigarettes, but he never wanted to go out. He even stopped seeing his psychologist, Dr. Milner. I was less concerned about him leaving therapy and more worried that he rarely left the house.

Besides bars on Saturday night and '80s Dance Night on Thursday, most of my social life revolved around academics. There were a handful of coffee shops that I went to on a nightly basis. My best friend Hannah and I would use that time to study and do our homework. It was something we held each other to every night so that we could get our work done and make sure we finished up our degrees in four years. Most of our friends dropped out before their junior year or had been in school six years without finishing a degree. We were determined not to fall into those categories. I was working toward a degree in English, and Hannah studied psychology.

Pat and I made an hourly wage and went into the office whenever we weren't in class. Just clerks, we relieved executives of tedious things, but we often found ourselves with nothing to do. We would download video games onto our computers, usually arcade games. Despite how hard I tried, I just couldn't beat Pat's high scores. I would introduce him to a game I had played for months, and he'd immediately destroy my record. He was always thinking a few steps ahead, taking a lot into account with each move. I always thought, "Well, he was always better at Nintendo, too," as if boys just have some built-in superiority when it comes to video games. Many of these games are very popular today—even our parents play them—but no one plays like he did.

He also spent a great deal of time at his desk writing e-mails, usually to our father. Raised in a conservative family, once he got to college Pat became very liberal. Something would happen in the news and it meant everything to Pat. It validated his feelings about this or that and dashed any claim otherwise. Honestly, it made me feel ignorant. I was so seldom aware of current events and was rarely moved by them.

As he worked out his new ideals about politics, he would debate them with our father. I liked to stay out of these conversations. I didn't know enough to talk politics. With Pat and Dad it was an intellectual melee. If Pat couldn't speak to Dad because he was busy or away from the office, Pat would write epic-length e-mails to him on his ideas. I'm not even sure Dad read those tomes. I think he just saw it in his inbox and came over to Pat's office to talk.

I was beginning to feel very closed-minded and shallow when I spoke to my brother. He was doing something very important. He was considering the whole and how every decision spirals out, affecting others and influencing other decisions. He was talking about Rwanda, politics in Tibet, the Shinto religion and how it affected World War II. He was taking in the history and the present moment of his whole world, not just his immediate surroundings, and trying to form an opinion that made a difference. He was growing, learning, and becoming a happier person. I thought the direction he was headed in was to one day make an impact and that he would use his ideas to make the world a better place on some scale no matter how small. At the same time, he was growing more and more introverted. He didn't want to meet new people or even socialize with old friends. He didn't like to use the phone anymore, and I found myself having to call his customers for him at work.

Everything I was ever taught about the economy in my little southern town was that fiscal conservatism was the only way to keep our heads above water. I didn't know anything else and never took the time to form my own opinion. My friends and professors were mostly liberal, but the majority of my classmates and coworkers were conservative. So when Pat would ask me about an issue, I felt tongue-tied. It didn't matter to him if I agreed with him, but he did seem particularly hurt that I never wondered about national or global issues. He would always say, "Think about it, Sarah. Just take some time and think."

Until then, I never thought about foreign relations, unions, the EPA, the ACLU, homeland security, or incarceration rates. My brother encouraged me to step outside myself, be mindful, to see the whole picture and empathize. Years later I would know the political issues that were truly important to me. By then Pat would be psychotic and have no interest in stepping into a voting booth.

We didn't live together long before I started to notice unhealthy changes in Pat's behavior. He didn't smoke weed anymore because his supplier was forty miles away at his former college. But he started drinking every night. Before, drinking had been something Pat did socially. He didn't keep much alcohol in his apartment, and I never noticed him drinking on a daily basis. When we moved in together, we bought a case of beer, and by the next morning most of it was gone. Pat would either restock the beer or come home with whiskey and Coke. Not only was I concerned, but I also felt responsible. That first case of beer had been my idea.

We had agreed to split all the utility expenses. After six months, Pat was consistently unable to play his half of the bills. He said he didn't have enough in his checking account, but he didn't appear to be spending more money than usual. While we didn't make much, I always had enough in my account. I would pay the bills myself, and he would promise to reimburse me when he got another paycheck. By the time he'd write me a check, the bills were piling up again. It was unfair and frustrating. For the first time, Pat was bad with money.

One day I walked into the office and my mother handed me some of Pat's mail that had been delivered to her house, his last residence. The letters were from his bank. He had been penalized because the balance of his checking account was less than twenty dollars. She paid the fee, but she was obviously concerned about it.

"Don't look at me. I'm the one paying the bills month after month."

"What's he buying?" Mom asked.

"I don't know. Same stuff he always buys, DVDs and music." Our paychecks were identical. If he bought something significant, I would have seen it. If he bought drugs, I would have smelled it or noticed his intoxication. I knew how much he drank, and he couldn't have spent it all on beer. I couldn't understand where it was all going and probably never will.

"Well, he's making enough to have more than twenty dollars in his account," Mom huffed. These were things that Mom or Dad would tell me but usually didn't broach with Pat. It was the same mismanagement of communication—communication deviance—that existed when we were kids. They were uncomfortable talking to Pat about it directly. They didn't want me to talk to him and patch it up instead, although it often felt like that was the expectation. They just wanted to vent for a moment and then move on, dissatisfied but letting it slide.

I knew Pat didn't want to lean on me when it came to expenses, but he continued to do so month to month. When I would press him to be more responsible with his money, he shrugged me off as if it was just standard nagging. I told him I was concerned about his drinking, and all he had to say was that he wasn't very happy lately.

I asked if he thought about going back to his psychologist, but he didn't seem interested. Although he liked Dr. Milner, Pat said he couldn't afford to see him on a weekly basis. This was a rupture in their therapeutic relationship. Despite the fact that Pat didn't even earn minimum wage and Dr. Milner had a sliding scale for payment, he insisted that Pat pay based on our father's salary.

"But you're an adult. Why does it matter what our parents make?" I was confused.

"That's what I told him. Then he said, 'Your father should be paying for this.'"

"What? Why?"

Pat just shrugged and chuckled.

"How does he even know what Dad makes?"

"He doesn't, not really. He just assumed based on things I said in therapy."

I shook my head. "That's screwed up, Pat." Now how could I ask him to see Dr. Milner again? "Aren't there other doctors in his practice? Maybe you could get a referral."

"That's a good idea," he perked up. "I'd like to see a psychiatrist, someone who could prescribe me something." He still believed that there was going to be a magic pill that would erase all his anxiety. Something that bothered him about seeing a psychologist was that Dr. Milner had to refer him to a physician for medication. In order to get the recommended antidepressant Milner suggested, Pat had to follow up with an MD.

If he felt that seeing a psychiatrist was going to make life easier, I was happy with that. I pictured Pat coming home with Prozac and a blissful smile on his face.

I wasn't sure when he had the appointment, but he said Dr. Barry Hollis was maybe in his thirties, much younger than Dr. Milner. He felt more comfortable talking to him. "That was the thing with Milner. He was always trying to be a father figure to me."

"Isn't he seventy years old?"

"Sixty-five, seventy."

"Grandfather figure," I joked.

"Dr. Hollis isn't so Freudian. He listened to me without thinking everything has something to do with Dad."

I wondered how old we'd have to be before we had to take responsibility for our lives, before we were unable to pin it on something our parents did. I also saw Dr. Milner for a short time, hoping he could help me with my anxiety. He never diagnosed me with anxiety disorder or depression. I received no formal diagnosis at all. When I told him I felt anxious or depressed, he would say, "That's perfectly normal considering the kind of family you grew up in." He seemed more interested in validating my feelings and combing through my past than he was in diagnosing me or talking about ways to alleviate my issues. I found it exhausting. He'd ask me to elaborate on some time in my adolescence, and I would spend an hour rehashing things that I considered unimportant. Then I wrote him a check. I went into therapy with a serious attitude, but I often went home feeling sapped of all my energy. Eventually I stopped keeping my appointments.

It's funny—in therapy you talk about what your parents did; you don't talk about their proclivities or gene expression. We never considered social anxiety as an inherited trait. It wasn't until much later, on my own, that I considered whether our parents had similar problems. Mom, like me, has never liked going to new places alone. She plans simple tasks out to a tee so they can be performed just right. Like most introverts, I like having a small, close group of friends rather than big parties and lots of strangers. My Dad is the same way. In fact, both of my parents would be happiest spending the night in, doing something solitary or with a few close friends. By nature we seem like an introverted family, and with that sometimes comes anxiety about social events and public scrutiny. I suppose in some cases anxiety can be taken to extremes; other times, being introverted is not pathological and is just a personality trait, a way of interacting or not interacting with the world.

Pat never really talked to me about what his psychiatrist thought of his symptoms. I found a prescription on the counter for a drug I had never heard of. Pat admitted it was a fairly new drug used to treat anxiety and depression associated with bipolar disorder.

"Wait a second. Dr. Hollis diagnosed you with bipolar disorder?"

"He didn't exactly say 'I diagnose you bipolar,' but he did say that it's used to treat bipolar disorder."

I gasped, "And what do you think about that?"

"He's the doctor, Sarah." He didn't offer more than that. I looked up the symptoms online and felt utterly confused. Bipolar is a mood disorder in which one constantly vacillates between high moods (happiness or irritability) and low (depressed) moods. There are two types of bipolar, the difference being the severity of the highs and lows. They were also broken up into classifications by whichever kind of episode the patient had most recently. From what I could gather, symptoms across the board looked like those in table 8.1.

I had never noticed any signs of depression before. There was no fatigue, no irritability or loss of pleasure in old activities. He had lost a great deal of weight since beginning college, but that was slowly, over the course of years.

Table 8.1. Symptoms of Bipolar Disorder

Manic symptoms:
- Persistent elevated, expansive, or irritable mood
- Grandiosity
- Extremely talkative, often speaking rapidly, flying from one subject to the next (called *pressured speech*)
- Decreased need for sleep
- Easily distracted by irrelevant thoughts
- Flight of ideas
- Highly productive, goal oriented
- Engaging in a great deal of pleasurable activities with high risks (e.g., spending sprees)

Major depressive symptoms:
- Persistent depressed mood
- Decreased pleasure in activities one used to enjoy
- Eating problems (loss of appetite or overeating)
- Low self-esteem
- Trouble sleeping or sleeping too much
- Difficulty concentrating
- Thoughts of suicide

On the other hand, he was increasingly withdrawn and had trouble sleeping. I definitely hadn't witnessed an elevated mood in Pat. He was never elated unless he'd had a lot of coffee. He was on an even keel.

He had complained about attention problems before, but I always assumed he was just fishing for a psychostimulant prescription. Psychostimulants prescribed for people with attention deficit disorder often found their way into the hands of college students. They use it to stay up all night and write a term paper or study for a final exam. During college, Pat had bought the drug from a student with a prescription several times. It stimulates the brain in much the same way that cocaine or methamphetamine does. I thought he was after a high, a buzz.

Since he had never had attention problems, I didn't really consider the fact that he truly couldn't concentrate all of a sudden. I just assumed he couldn't stay glued to a book he needed to read for class because the book was boring. That happened to me all the time. No student wants to read and study everything you put in front of them. I thought he just needed to buckle down and muscle through it.

I wondered if the new drug he was taking was also a stimulant that would improve attention, but it wasn't. When I did an Internet search on the name, I found that the drug was an antipsychotic used to manage psychosis. I couldn't believe my eyes.

The side effects of the drug were serious: dizziness, blurred vision, weight gain, excessive saliva, and a rise in blood sugar, just to name a few. The prescription label warned against drinking while using the medication. I read that it was also prescribed for schizophrenia and had a rare side effect called tardive dyskinesia, a disorder that causes involuntary, repetitive body movements.

Why would a person not convinced that they have bipolar disorder or any other mental illness take such a serious medication? Obviously Pat's attention problems and social anxiety were mounting concerns for him, but I can't be sure what Pat might have said that resulted in Dr. Hollis prescribing an antipsychotic. Today I realize that the doctor's gut reaction was more accurate than we could have realized.

The first hitch in taking the medication was that it interfered with Pat's drinking habits. He tried doing both, but he felt extremely groggy. The antipsychotic increases the effects of alcohol. As Pat started to take the medication and continued to drink as much as he normally did, the result was sedation. One evening, he got up to use the bathroom, lost consciousness, and fell sideways onto the porcelain toilet. He hit it so hard that the toilet was moved from its base. He didn't tell me about it right away. I went to use the bathroom and discovered the damage myself.

When our parents saw the broken toilet weeks later they were confused and angry, but they didn't press Pat about it. All he offered was that he had gotten light-headed and fell. Then they turned to me for further explanation. I said that Pat was very thin and didn't eat much. It made sense he would have low blood pressure and dizzy spells.

After breaking the toilet, Pat used the medication less than prescribed. He continued to drink every day but took the antipsychotic only sometimes.

I arrived home one evening to find him sitting on the sofa looking at his feet. "What are you doing?"

"What does this look like to you?" He pointed to his foot. There were faint red patches on his skin.

"What did you do?"

"I didn't do anything. It's on the other foot, too."

"Pat, are hives a side effect of your medication?"

He looked at me with raised eyebrows. "Maybe so."

"Don't scratch it," I warned. A quick search of the Internet turned up the rare allergic reaction. "It says to stop taking the medication immediately and contact your doctor."

At that point the hives were spreading. He now had blotchy shoulders and a few on his chest. "Will it go away?"

"It should, but if you start having trouble breathing or something we need to go to the hospital."

"So you're saying I shouldn't go smoke a cigarette?"

I sighed. "Give it an hour, at least."

The hives cleared up. Without consulting Dr. Hollis about it, he stopped taking the medication entirely.

As the spring semester came to a close and he had difficulty studying for exams, he made another appointment with Dr. Hollis. This time he came home with Adderall. Once again he denied being formally diagnosed by the doctor but said that they had "discussed" attention deficit disorder. He got through finals and enrolled in a summer semester. He only had two courses left before he would graduate.

He went through a month's supply of Adderall in ten days. It's an upper, and I figured he just wanted the rush. I never considered that he was upping the dosage to get the same effect that a person with attention deficit disorder might. Looking back, Pat's social anxiety wasn't the only red flag missed. I responded to his complaints about attention with eye rolling.

One day, I came home to the television blaring and music playing on the stereo in the living room. Pat was on the couch with a book in his lap. He was trying to read.

"How can you concentrate with all this on?"

"I couldn't concentrate when they were off. Nothing else was working." He didn't look up from his book. "I'm trying something new."

He was acting strange, but what was worse was the way he offered so little by way of explanation. Later I noticed one of his books open on the kitchen table. The margins were scribbled with notes, arrows pointed at this and that, and most of the paragraphs were highlighted in their entirety. Every page was a mess. Most of the notations were simply hand-copied sentences of the text right next to it. He gave me his old paperbacks all the time, and I'd never seen him do this to a book before. Things were strange enough that I could not deny that something was off about Pat.

Without the Adderall, I'm not sure he would have finished his bachelor of arts in philosophy. He defended his thesis on empiricist David Hume's theory of causation. I didn't understand any of it, although I proofread it for him. In summer 2005, he didn't attend his graduation ceremony. His diploma was sent to our house. Our parents felt cheated out of getting to see him walk in the ceremony. It meant something to them after all this time. I hadn't considered it, and I don't think Pat did either. At that point he was just happy to be finished with school, although his books were still piled high on our kitchen table.

He had been such a tidy teenager. His room was much cleaner than mine. I had stacks of books and papers all over my room. It was difficult to navigate without tripping over something. I collected half-empty soda cans. I didn't throw them out until there was a stack of about ten on my desk. I never did laundry, and eventually my Mom would offer to throw mine in with hers. The clutter was organized in such a way that only I knew where to find anything. Pat, on the other hand, made his bed every day. His things were always put away, with nothing left on the floor or dresser. His garbage can was usually empty. He washed his clothes regularly. I can't say he was remarkably clean. Things were usually dusty or dust-bunnied, and while he showered every day, there were always marks on his white door from his hands. Mom said he had always had dirty hands since he was a little boy. It was like he just didn't notice they were dirty.

While we were living together, Pat was anything but tidy. His things were all over the house. He didn't put anything away after he was finished with it. Schoolbooks littered the living room. His bedroom was a sea of clothing and papers. He'd set up recording equipment in the kitchen, and the table would be encumbered for months. We had one of our dogs living there with us, an older female boxer. She shed like crazy, even with daily brushing. The fur doubled the need to clean the place on a regular basis. Come Sunday, I'd have to nag Pat to help me. Sometimes he'd say that he had to do yard work, so I should do the housework. The only time I could count on him to pitch in was if our parents were coming over.

Besides having lost the good cleaning habits he once had, Pat began sleeping in the living room every night. At first I was sure he'd just fallen asleep watching a movie, but there he was every night thereafter. It made it difficult to come and go as I pleased, and even more difficult to get a glass of water at night without disturbing him.

He didn't deal with most people in person. I sympathized with his feelings. Calling strangers was a harrowing experience for me too. At this time, I was reveling in the boom of online shopping. More people were using e-mail and other social media than ever. It was like the world was finally embracing my introverted tendencies. Not having to interact face-to-face with a person always brought great relief to me. If I have the option to e-mail or chat online, I'll do that rather than phone someone.

Pat usually ran his own errands, but he would put them off until the eleventh hour, when he absolutely needed something. Sometimes he'd ask me to bring him something, but I didn't like to encourage that. Before I knew it, he was asking me to bring him a whole list of groceries. I nearly ran out of reasons as to why he should get them himself.

Pat didn't seem to get much joy out of being with his friends anymore. He didn't even go to concerts. With my friends, he was standoffish. He came off as gruff, all business. I would explain, "Don't worry. He's not angry or anything. He's just like that."

One weekend, Hannah's boyfriend was in from out of town. He was a funny guy with a dry sense of humor. She brought him over to my house, and we sat around smoking cigarettes on the back porch, joking around. I introduced him to Pat, and they got on really well. Hannah and I were both really pleased to see him interacting, laughing and smiling. The air of seriousness was gone.

I realized we suddenly had thousands of channels in the living room. He had upgraded the cable so he would have unlimited viewing options. When he wasn't watching TV he was playing video games. One was an action role-playing game called *Fable*. The idea was that you lived in this medieval-type kingdom and you were training to become a warrior. Decisions you made in the game would decide if you would eventually turn out to be good or evil. But it was more or less an endless game. You could perform a million different tasks and challenges alongside actions that would eventually lead to the conclusion of the game. It seemed to me to be another world, and Pat liked to stay there and experiment with it most of the time.

When he went to sleep, I noticed that he would stack all the throw pillows on the love seat and then sleep on the longer couch. There was a method to it. The pillows had to be in the same position every night. In the morning he'd get in the shower, and I'd put the pillows back. Sometimes they just stayed in the pile night after night.

"I gave up the big room, and you sleep in the den every night."

"You want to switch rooms?" He dragged on his cigarette.

I didn't care about the rooms. I just wanted to understand what was going on. "No, I just—what's with the pillows?"

He shrugged and flicked the cigarette. I couldn't tell if he was hiding something or if there really was no significance to the stacking of the pillows.

"You know, it's hard to do stuff at night with you sleeping in the living room."

"I don't go to bed until like midnight."

"But I feel like I'll disturb you."

"You don't disturb me," he said tersely and got up to go inside.

I sat on the back porch listening to the cicadas while he went back to his video game. Things felt dark and confusing. Maybe we just weren't ready to be adults living on our own or something else was legitimately tinkering with the formula. Something wasn't right anymore.

There were many times that I felt my brother wasn't forthcoming with me. When he wouldn't answer for changes in his behavior, he felt like a perfect stranger to me. He had always shared with me what was going on. I kicked myself for making light when he had moments of introspection. One night he was drinking and he turned to me and said, "Remember when we were young and I used to make fun of you for writing in journals?"

"Yeah. And my poetry."

He chuckled slightly. "That was messed up. You were just—being you, being creative. That's who you were. And I was a dick about it. I don't know why. That must have been hard."

I shrugged and nodded, smoking my cigarette. All that stuff was behind me. I didn't think about it, and it hadn't discouraged me. I still wrote every day. But something about the way I reacted made Pat feel stonewalled.

"Are you listening to me?"

"Yeah, Pat. I agreed with you," I said brusquely.

"Jesus Christ. Don't you care? I'm trying to apologize." I remember the look on his face. I can hear those words clearly even today. Was it the beginning of the end? Was it then he decided to shut me out?

I sat back in my patio chair, the dingy cushion clinging to my legs. The heat in August in New Orleans creeps into your pores. I smoked and thought about the days when I lived with Maw-Maw Alice. Lighthearted overnights with Pat. The three of us sitting around and making fun of each other, or mostly just making fun of me. Going through my sociology books trying to figure out how and where he learned so much and I hadn't. Introducing him to *Yellow Submarine*, the cartoon, and assuring him, "Yes, this really is just that trippy." Those days felt different than these. Something ominous hung over us, casting a shadow over my heart. I second-guessed my feelings. I spoke to my best friend Hannah about it, but none of it made sense to either of us. I knew something was brewing, but I didn't dare say it. I was about to start my senior year of college, and I had little stress to spare. But something else was headed right for us, something that couldn't be put on the back burner, something that would change our lives forever. A category 5 hurricane nearly five hundred miles in diameter named Katrina was making her way for New Orleans at 175 miles per hour.

9

Hurricane Katrina and a Broken Mind

Just a month after Pat's summer graduation, Hannah's boyfriend came to town again for another visit before fall classes started up. I arranged to have them over again, thinking that it would be a pick-me-up for Pat. Hannah said her boyfriend was looking forward to seeing him too. But the night they came over to the house, Pat would barely even look at them. He spent all his time in his bedroom, coming out only to smoke cigarettes. His salutations were barely even nods. He'd plow through the cigarette in two minutes and then go back inside. I apologized to them, "I really don't know what's up with him. He drinks all night and crashes on the couch in the living room."

I was getting fed up with Pat. I could sympathize with his *quirks* during times of stress, like when he was taking finals. But all that was over now, and he wasn't returning to baseline. He rarely socialized. He didn't even want to call our clients when we were at work, a responsibility that was then heaped on me. He was drinking heavily on a daily basis as if he was trying to run or hide from something. He wouldn't share with me what he went looking for at the bottom of the wine bottle. He did tell me that he had stopped taking the Adderall, but that gave me little comfort. I don't think he wanted to stop using the drug, but rather he simply didn't want to keep his appointments with the psychiatrist in order to get refill prescriptions.

I was about to begin the fall semester of my senior year of college. I registered carefully, making sure I'd be able to get the right sequence of remaining credits so I'd be out in the spring. Classes started August 22, and while I hustled off to campus, I envied Pat who got to stay in our air-conditioned office all day. With highs over ninety degrees Fahrenheit, August in Louisiana is arguably the hottest and most humid month.

That Thursday some girlfriends held game night; we were burning off our last days before schoolwork picked up and midterms started breathing down our necks. I remember complaining because other universities weren't holding classes until the following week. I went home early because I had a class the next morning. Sitting in lecture, my professor warned that we might have to change some of the due dates for assignments assuming we wouldn't be holding class on Monday.

"Why not?" asked those of us awake enough to be cognizant.

"Because of the hurricane," a girl said.

"What hurricane?" another student asked.

"The one all the way out by Florida?" I asked.

"That's not even a hurricane. It's a tropical storm," someone in the back called.

My teacher took control of the floor again. "Look, just be mindful it could head this way. Listen to the radio." Then she continued the lecture.

The last I had heard of this hurricane, it was out by Key West. How could they know its path would bring it all the way out to New Orleans?

There weren't many students on campus that day. It was baffling. Usually the first week of school is nothing but lines, traffic jams, and litter. Then a couple of weeks later it calms down.

I left campus around 1:00 p.m., and when I got to work I learned that the governor of Louisiana had declared a state of emergency. It was hard to wrap my head around. Just yesterday this storm was nothing to us, and now it was the Big One. People were going home early from work, talking about evacuating. My dad gave me an earnest look and asked what we wanted to do.

Pat didn't have anything to say. He was reading an e-mail on his computer. It was as if he didn't care.

"I'm not going anywhere," I said. I sat down in my chair and continued to work until five o'clock.

Katrina wasn't the first time in 2005 that people in southeast Louisiana had evacuated. Many also left in July, when a category 1 storm named Cindy pushed through. Cindy hit Grand Isle and just knocked out some power along the coast. We were back to work the next day. But at some point forecasters had said Cindy would get bigger and stronger, and when she hit New Orleans head on, it would be the Big One. Everyone knew about the Big One, the perfect storm, the worst-case scenario. The day the Big One comes, the levees will fail; the storm surge will push water into Lake Pontchartrain north of New Orleans and it will top the levees. The city will become a cereal bowl. Everything will be gone.

But every storm was the Big One. Every forecasted track had a hurricane headed right for us, and yet it never landed just right. Every time we evacuated we spent tons of money on storm preparations, gasoline, and hotel rooms. We sat in endless traffic waiting to get out and again waiting to get home. We lost money. Kids missed school. And all for nothing. Because officials would rather be safe than sorry, they almost always tell us to leave. But you hear people who grew up here telling the honest truth: "It's just a category 1. We're not going anywhere."

Besides, without a real test of their strength, the average citizen had no reason to doubt the strength of our levee system or pumping stations. The wetlands south of New Orleans were depleting, and we had lost a very important buffer between our homes and the strongest hurricane-force winds. But without a real test, anyone who wasn't an engineer, a marine scientist, or a meteorologist would never guess that every single thing that could go wrong on August 29, 2005, would go wrong.

That weekend the storm followed its track straight to our front door. Sunday, August 28, before Katrina made landfall, Dad finally convinced me to leave. I could hear the fear in his voice, and I knew it wasn't like the others. It was bigger. Trudging through the warm Gulf water, it was getting stronger.

He drove across Lake Pontchartrain to get us and take us to stay with him and Mom. Riding in one car worked best because the traffic out of the city was so bad it took us five hours to make a forty-five-minute trip. We would ride out the storm together in Covington, just forty miles north of the city. Heavily forested, Saint Tammany Parish is higher ground. I had no idea at the time, but it would mean everything to be with my family after Katrina hit. If I hadn't been with them, if I had stayed in New Orleans, my parents would not have been able to find out if I was okay for weeks, maybe over a month.

Pat was happy to evacuate if it made Dad feel more comfortable. He wasn't worried and agreed we'd probably be back home by the middle of the week.

We packed for just a few days. I brought my homework. I had to read Henry James's *The Turn of the Screw* by Thursday.

Passing through town, everything was empty and boarded up. We hit traffic at the bridge and crawled from that point forward. At the foot of the Causeway toll bridge that spans twenty-four miles across Lake Pontchartrain, there is a hotel. I watched it slowly recede from my view over the course of many hours sitting in traffic. I remember the grave look on the face of every driver around us. The storm coverage on the radio was disheartening. I held my breath, wondering if it was really happening.

When we reached the house, Mom was cooking everything in the refrigerator and freezer. The kitchen counter was a smorgasbord of chicken tenders, deer tamales, and red beans and rice. The floor was a maze of ice chests. She looked relieved to see us.

I put my bags in my old bedroom, and Pat did the same. Dad took a walk around the yard to survey the trees and judge how close they would come to hitting the house, as if we could do anything about it now. There were pine trees everywhere, one hundred feet high with taproots from thirty-five to seventy-five feet below the ground. Would they hold in one-hundred-mile-per-hour wind?

Mom and Dad called around to find out where everyone had evacuated to. I spoke to friends on the phone, even ex-boyfriends I hadn't heard from in years. Everyone had gotten out to Shreveport, Montgomery, Houston, Dallas, Jackson, or Natchez. Pat didn't call anyone. He smoked cigarettes on the porch and played with the dogs.

Pat and I would change the TV from news to movies. We were done watching footage of past storms and seeing images of the empty French Quarter on the Weather Channel. Part of me just couldn't take all the doomsday stuff seriously. The news didn't sound any different than when Cindy came through. The storm was big, but it could have been faster. How warm could the Gulf really be? Bathwater? How could that be? Didn't President Bush say that scientists were divided on the issue of global warming and were undecided whether warming was actually happening at all?

The wind woke me up the morning of the storm. I had several missed calls. The power was already out. I found Mom in the kitchen. Dad and Pat were on the back porch.

"I thought we weren't supposed to go outside during a hurricane." I had heard that my whole life.

"The way the wind moves, it goes around the porch. You can't feel it." The back porch was located on a corner of the house. They were standing in the nook, wearing raincoats, watching the pine trees bend, billow, and part.

"Are you sure it's okay?"

"Sarah, they'll come in if it gets too bad."

Standing by the kitchen window, Dad gestured for me to come out. I pulled on a hooded sweatshirt and opened the door slowly. The wind was endless white noise. He gestured for me to stay against the wall of the house. If I reached out my arm the wind and rain would get me, but it couldn't touch me there.

"Some pine trees have come down," he shouted over the wind.

Pat pointed at one, but I couldn't make it out in the rain.

"The whole tree?"

"No, they snap in half!"

"Right down the middle," Pat said.

Dad pointed to the woods behind the house as a new sound filled the air. It was getting closer. The pine trees waved violently as the gust barreled through.

Rain drops in that wind seemed small as crumbs, but if one hit you, it was like a shard of glass. They dotted the porch along with leaves, flowers, and grass, everything torn to bits.

We heard a loud pop and looked around nervously for the tree. Dad looked around the corner of the porch, shielding his eyes from the debris.

"It was over there." Pat pointed across the yard, far away from the house.

Then there was a new sound, not like the last. It sounded like crumbling stone. Without a word, Dad instinctively grabbed me by the middle of my sweatshirt, opened the back door, and threw me inside.

"What was that?" Mom asked.

"I don't know. We heard something weird."

She rushed to the door as Dad and Pat came inside. "Sorry about that, it sounded close to the house."

"What was it?"

"The old oak tree, it fell to pieces."

Never healthy since we lived there, the old oak was ancient. It sat at the foot of the pond, barely alive.

"It was all rotten inside," Mom explained.

"It sounded so much closer to the house." I was frightened, but I went back outside for at least an hour. When the winds died down, the rain fell more heavily. Then it was over. We saw it come, and we saw it go. I eventually took a nap in the living room, waiting for life to get back to normal. When I got up, the sun was out. I sat in a chair by the pool, the water still, the pump unable to run without power. I finished *The Turn of the Screw*, and Pat told me about Henry James's brother, the philosopher William James.

"Like us," I said, "writer and philosopher."

He just made his usual brief hint of a smile. I told him he could borrow the book after I finished my English class.

With the power out, we ate cold food from the ice chests, hoping we'd be able to get more ice by the time what we had melted. There was no escaping the ninety-degree heat, so we opened all the windows. "We're living like our ancestors. New Orleans didn't always have air conditioning, you know."

"I know, Dad." I rolled my eyes. I didn't want to live like my ancestors.

As night fell, the air circulating made it bearable inside. I slept on an old sofa in the living room because it had a cold green marble floor that called to me. Pat slept on the other sofa in the living room, just as he had the night before.

"He said he doesn't need a bed," Mom told me.

"See, I told you that's what he does. He won't sleep in his bed at home either. He always sleeps on the sofa. He piles up pillows on the love seat in this very specific pattern."

"Oh, Sarah," Mom shook her head. She didn't seem to think any of that was important.

I woke up Tuesday morning to someone rubbing my arm. "You better get up, baby girl," Dad said. "The levees broke."

Water had been pouring into New Orleans all night. I sat down on the back porch in my pajamas and lit a cigarette. A man on the radio was talking to a woman in the Bywater. She was in her attic. Her flooded street was, as she said, "flowing like a river." She asked the DJ for help. "If there's any NOPD or fire or rescue teams listening, please, please—" The call cut off.

It went on like that all morning. Callers constantly asked, "Where is FEMA? Where is the Red Cross?" The Coast Guard rescued people off one roof; meanwhile phone calls came into the radio station from five more people trapped in their homes. I wondered how they were even getting a call out. Our landline was down, and our cell phones had no signal; the towers were down.

As the day pushed forward and nothing improved, it dawned on me that it was over. Presidents of the lower parishes reported that we were not allowed to return home. They said it was unsafe and roadways had to be inspected. Anyone heading into the New Orleans metro area would be turned away by the National Guard. They didn't say when we could go home again. Then it hit me. Wondering when we would get power again was silly. I should be thinking about whether or not I would even finish college that year. Would the school even reopen? Would teachers come back? What about doctors, prescriptions, daycares, jobs, gasoline, and everything else? They didn't even have clean water; the water supply was contaminated and required boiling before use.

We had well water. We heated it over a propane BBQ pit so we could make instant coffee. While we listened to the radio, shaking our heads, Pat was walking around the yard. He gathered broken branches and dragged them over to a burn pile. Everything was too green, it would be weeks before it would burn, and that was if the rain held off. He did it anyway. Some branches were so big they had to be rolled. Dad got up to help him and told him he didn't have to do that right now. Pat seemed indifferent, unemotional. He wasn't worried about what was happening in New Orleans. He was matter-of-fact about everything, as if he'd expected it. The rest of us were in shock.

With no response from FEMA, life in New Orleans was on hold and deteriorating. At some point the DJ mentioned people rescued from New Orleans East being dropped off on the UNO campus. They weren't given any water or food, so they broke into vending machines. For shelter overnight, they tried to break into buildings. I looked down at *The Turn of the Screw* and gave a halfhearted laugh. Pat came over to the porch to smoke a cigarette, and I told him, "I read all that for nothing. That class is canceled indefinitely. Who knows when I'll get to finish school."

"Jesus, Sarah. Stop thinking about yourself." He was curt, although he showed no sign of being angry or annoyed. I couldn't tell if he didn't know he had hurt my feelings or if he just didn't care.

"Are you serious?" I studied his blank face. "You're not worried about anything right now? You're not worried that they're telling us we can't go home?"

He sipped his coffee and shrugged.

"Pat, your city is drowning. Everything you know has changed forever. You're not thinking about that right now? Things will never be the same."

He puffed the cigarette all the way down in a heartbeat and pinched the last burning ashes out onto the ground. He'd started doing this recently. "I'm going to finish cleaning up the yard." He started back toward the burn pile. I watched him walk away, his shirt clinging to the sweat on his back. I remember thinking for the first time in that very instant, "This is not my brother. I do not know this person."

We stayed at our parents' house without electricity, running water, or phone service for three weeks. The two bathtubs had been filled before the storm, so we used them to bathe until they were so full of soap the water was thick and covered in a layer of foam. Sometimes I would swim in the now green swimming pool just to get that clean, chlorine smell. Pat may not have bathed the whole time.

At night we all sat on the back porch, drinking beers by lamplight and listening to the radio. As the news became more positive, the sense of urgency became feelings of regret. We should have expected this perfect storm. If we go back, are we putting our whole lives at risk again? I couldn't handle the fact that everything had gone wrong during Katrina and no one was taking responsibility. We even heard other Americans on the radio say they shouldn't rebuild our city if it's under sea level. I argued with my Dad, "We shouldn't live in a place that could be taken away from us in a second."

"But what about San Francisco and all the cities in Tornado Alley? What about St. Louis? Fire has taken out whole cities, too," Dad said.

"Nobody helped us. Another storm will wash New Orleans away completely, and we'll be left to fend for ourselves again."

"Next time, hopefully we will have learned from those mistakes," Dad said.

I was doubtful, and my eyes welled with tears. Pat drank his beer and didn't seem the least bit interested in our conversation.

"It's going to be all right." Mom squeezed my shoulder.

"We'll get it straightened out," Dad nodded.

I received a few text messages from friends days after they sent them. I responded, but it took days to get those messages through as well. Telegrams would have been more efficient. Over the course of several days texting my best friend Hannah, we came to the conclusion that we would lose that semester and finish school late the next year. It was a hard reality to face, but at least we weren't alone. We knew people who left the state and enrolled in other schools free of charge for the semester, but we felt bound to stay with our families.

It was nearly October when we went home. Thankfully our house had no wind or water damage. By then the power was back on. Many of our neighbors had roof damage. Trees had smashed up porches, pools, and attics. The flood picked up sharp little things from everywhere and left them in the street. So many people got flat tires that auto shops all over town ran out of stock.

Dad's office got a couple of feet of water. The lower floor was gutted, and the second floor was refurnished to house the whole office. Now we just had to wait for everyone to return to the office so we could all begin working again. Of course many never returned. That meant twice as much work for the remaining employees. We were so short staffed at one point that job titles meant nothing; everyone did everything. We faced it bravely because we had no other choice. We smoked twice as many cigarettes as before. Standing on the second-floor balcony one afternoon, I estimated based on what was left in my pack that I had gone out to smoke at least ten times that day. I skipped lunch.

Across the street from the office several apartment buildings also had extensive roof damage. Shingles and even roofing tacks littered the grass and sidewalks. Migrant workers from Texas were hired by most contractors. They spoke only Spanish. While we smoked on the balcony, Pat listened to them intently. He had taken Spanish for several years in school, but he didn't know enough to make out anything but the odd word here and there. It didn't matter, he said; he was sure they were talking about us. Based on past experience, I assumed he thought they were catcalling and flirting with me. I didn't think so and shrugged it off.

A week later, our neighbors hired several Mexican roofers to reshingle their house. I noticed that Pat wouldn't smoke on the back porch if they were out there working. He said he could hear them talking about him. "Pat, they speak Spanish. You don't know what they're talking about."

"Then why are they always looking at me?"

"They can't even see you. All they can see is the patio roof."

He huffed and dismissed me. I knew I didn't convince him, and he didn't want to talk to me about it anymore. Once he sensed I didn't agree, he'd just keep his feelings from me.

I understand the suspicion of being observed and judged by strangers. It's common in social anxiety. Having to walk through a room full of people is a harrowing experience. You're so self-conscious that you can't imagine that onlookers are thinking about anything but you, the way you look and how you're all wrong. It takes a great deal of work to realize that they're thinking about you about as much as you think about the strangers who pass by you every day, which is to say very little.

It was unlikely, but perhaps the roofers were looking at Pat. How could I know? But the fact that it unsettled him so was still bizarre. There's no crime in seeing a person. He seemed to think he was being made fun of, but there was nothing to poke fun at. What's funny about a very plain guy smoking on his porch?

When I spoke to Dad about this, he agreed that it was strange. His eyes were wide. I would grow accustomed to this response from people when I talked to them about Pat's behavioral changes. "What should I do?"

"You're sure he's not smoking weed or anything anymore?"

"I'm sure. I mean, it's highly unlikely."

Dad got quiet and shook his head. We left it at that. He didn't seem any more certain of what to do than I was.

I watched Pat and waited to see if things would change. Soon he wouldn't even talk if he was outside on the porch or in the yard. He would get aggravated with me, throw down his cigarette, and storm inside if I said something to him.

One weekend he was in the front yard mowing. He came in through the garage with an infuriated look on his face. "Someone just took my picture!" he told me angrily.

"What?" I was cleaning up in the kitchen.

He stood in the doorway, seething. "Somebody just drove by in a car and took my picture."

I couldn't understand his agitation. "Pat, people are taking pictures of storm damage all around town. People say even out-of-towners are coming to see the destruction," I explained honestly.

"There's no damage here!"

"Wait," I shook my head. "Was it the driver who took your picture?"

"No, somebody in the backseat."

"A kid?"

"How do I know?"

"What are you saying here? You think somebody intentionally took your picture?"

"Exactly."

"So what?"

"Why do they want my picture?"

"I don't know. People take pictures of all sorts of things. I have pictures of people I only met one time years ago. It's not uncommon. It's not unusual for somebody to just be playing with their camera while they ride in a car. It's not a crime."

He looked at me suspiciously, as if I was lying to him.

"What?" I asked in disbelief. I was so confused. Never one to call him names, I kept myself from saying he was being stubborn and unreasonable.

He said no more but was still fuming when he went back outside to finish mowing. I started to clean again. Then I began to think about the traffic on our street—lots of cars, speeding away. Could someone really take a picture that quickly? Could he even see it as they drove by? I dropped the rag I was holding and looked back at the door to the garage he had just gone through. In that moment I finally realized that he wasn't just misinterpreting things around him; he was telling me about things that were not real.

When I told my friends about it, they didn't think much of it. People said there was probably a good explanation, but they couldn't offer one. Some suggested maybe someone did take pictures of him. I agreed that it was possible, but it still didn't explain how angry and suspicious it made him.

I related the incident to Mom and Dad. Dad's eyes were wide and wary again, but Mom just shrugged. She said that because she wasn't there to see it for herself, she couldn't be sure of what Pat was thinking. "It's not necessarily anything to worry about."

"Well, I've seen the pillow thing for myself. I know that's something," Dad reminded her. "I think I have it figured out. The way he stacks them on the love seat just so blocks the view from the front porch. You can't see anything, just pillows. I saw it myself when I came over early in the morning and he was still asleep."

"What should I do?" I asked again.

"There's nothing we can do," Dad said. "Hopefully it's temporary."

"Yes, maybe he's just stressed," Mom suggested wishfully.

Later that month, Pat was fired from the office. I wasn't present when it happened, but I got both sides of the story. Dad asked Pat to do something, and he flatly refused. Dad asked again, and Pat stood up and angrily told him, "No, I won't."

Dad was flabbergasted. He asked me what I thought was going on. I told him the explanation Pat gave me. "He said he saw you across the street talking to the Hispanic roofers."

"What?"

"He said this morning when he came into work he saw you across the street talking to the roofers and laughing."

"I spoke to the contractor this morning, but it was only for a second. What does it matter?"

"He thinks those people are talking about him. Colluding, conspiring."

He sat back in his chair and sighed.

"I told you something was wrong with him. I told you he was acting strange," I said. A prickle of anger sent my heart racing.

"I thought it was just the hurricane and all the crazy bullshit that was going on. He's not using drugs again, is he?"

"No," I said bitterly.

"Well, whatever is going on, whatever he's dealing with, it's better he's not here while he's doing it."

I glared out the office window. One less person to help at work sounded insurmountable. Furthermore, I seemed to be the only person concerned that Pat wasn't just going through some temporary rough time. I saw things escalating. He wasn't the man I knew anymore.

When I spoke to friends about it, at first they would make excuses for Pat's behavior. "Oh, he's probably just being funny." As it became more unusual, they wouldn't even try. They would look far off with big, scared eyes and shake their heads. I felt I had nowhere to turn. Then things seemed to level off. He stopped talking about the roofers next door, he calmed down about talking outdoors, and he even went to the movies. *Good Night, and Good Luck* (2005) was the last film he saw in a theater.

Pat started to look for work, interviewing at a local bank. It didn't go well. He described his interviewer as uppity. "He acted like he was doing me a favor even talking to me."

"Why did he even call you in if he was so unimpressed with your resume?"

"I don't know. Then he had this other guy come in, somebody in sales, which is what I was interviewing for. He was twice as rude. Fast talking. Full of shit."

"Do you really want to work in sales?"

"I don't know. It was just a possibility."

"If you want to do something with the philosophy degree, maybe you should go back to school." I always imagined Pat finding a career in academia.

"Maybe."

The next week he had out his old course catalogs looking at PhD programs at his alma mater, UNO. There was nothing for philosophy, but political science was a great interest for him. Because Katrina had flung professors hither and thither, they waved the recommendation requirement on his application. By December 2005, he was accepted into the political science PhD program for the spring term.

10

Abnormal Psychology and Unreturned Phone Calls

The Christmas after Katrina, in 2005, many of Pat's friends got together and went out in the French Quarter. I didn't believe he would actually go with them until I saw him leave the house. I even called him a few times that evening while I was out, wondering if he wanted to meet up. When I got home, he still wasn't back. He didn't return until the early morning.

He didn't seem like he wanted to talk about that night at first. Then it was all he would talk about. Apparently he met a girl while he was out. He spent all night competing with one of his friends for her attention. That's why he stayed out so late. The girl eventually went home alone.

He seemed a little bummed out that the girl wasn't interested in him, but much more concerned with how competitive he felt with his friend. "He's probably mad at me now," he said.

I didn't know what to tell him, and he wouldn't be swayed from the subject. It sounded like an uneventful night, and yet he couldn't let it go. The thoughts were pervasive. He'd talk about what he said, what he drank, where he went, and how he acted. He was so self-conscious that he was unable to cope with the idea that other people had been watching him and possibly judging him. He picked apart every little detail from that night, feeling insecure, wishing he could change it, asking for my feedback, and maybe even wishing he had never gone out at all. I was at a loss to help him. When I get hung up on a situation where I might have made a fool of myself, I have to distract myself.

I think about anything else, sometimes burying my nose in a book. I want to put time and space between that event and the present. I'm sure that rubbing my face in it over and over again isn't going to help me feel any more secure, but Pat can't always let those things go. It's almost as if the discomfort he feels convinces him there is something there in that memory that he must go over and analyze. But there is no answer. The past cannot be changed.

He only took a handful of graduate school classes before he dropped out of the political science program. He said it was too hard for him to concentrate on the material. Again I saw his textbooks scribbled with notes, arrows, and underlines. I couldn't make sense of his notations. One of the first topics discussed in lecture had been on the Patriot Act, under which the government could conduct wiretapping without a warrant. He told me, "See? Anyone could be listening to you when you use the phone." It was hard to argue with him. He was both right and wrong. Yet he wasn't concerned about his rights being violated; he was more interested in proving that other people could easily spy on him. After he dropped out of school, conversations about spying and about that Christmas night out finally stopped.

He finally seemed calm, maybe even a little depressed. But it was a welcome change. At least it seemed normal. I would have felt depressed in his shoes as well. It was much better than the suspicion and accusations since Katrina. He didn't seem anxious about being watched anymore. He went to bed at a normal hour, and often in his own bedroom instead of on the couch. But he did still have strange new habits that worried me.

Before he opened a bottle of wine in the evening, he followed a stringent routine. He would exercise vigorously on the treadmill, running seven to ten miles. He did this in the dark, with barely any light coming in from other rooms to see. I asked him why, and he said it made it easier to zone out and not worry about feeling tired. Soon he also began taking out his contacts so he truly couldn't see anything at all. If I came in the front door and switched on a light while he was on the treadmill, he'd be visibly annoyed with me. Thinking back on it now, that was something that came with onset. He was getting grumpier. Even more set in his ways than when we were teens, he didn't like to be questioned and often expected me to intuit his wishes.

After exercising, he made dinner. He usually ate only one meal, and it was the same meal every day—a bowl of salad with honey mustard dressing, a can of tuna, and fried wontons on top. He ate it standing in the same spot at the kitchen counter. Then he opened a bottle of wine and would often finish it by himself in front of the TV.

It was common to find milk or food left out on the counter all night. He would drink so much that he would have to eat something more. Sometimes he forgot the meal in the midst of making it. I'd find a bowl of cereal left out and beside it the unpoured milk. Other times I found my leftovers from the night before missing from the fridge. Pat never remembered eating these things and was therefore unapologetic. He said he'd gone to bed. Sleepwalking and night eating are common in schizophrenia, and it's something Pat does to this day.

I was thankful for the new sense of calm in the house, but it was impossible to ignore these quirky new developments. One evening I came home from studying at a coffee shop and found a printed poem I had written on my bed. It was late, and Pat was already in bed, so I asked him about it in the morning. He said a girl had come by to see me, and since I wasn't there, she had asked him to give me the poem. I managed to piece together what had happened. The poem had been published on the website of a literary journal. It was vaguely based on an ex-girlfriend. The girl who dropped it off was my ex's new girlfriend. I was furious with the intrusion and tore it up.

To my surprise the incident didn't play into Pat's suspicions at all. He was recently very suspicious of our neighbors if they were outside in their yard. If he heard anything outside, he would turn off the television or radio, stop whatever he was doing, and tiptoe to the nearest window to see what it was. He'd peek through the blinds. If there was a person out there, he would watch quietly for a half hour or more.

Yet the visit from the girl with the poem didn't stir him up at all. It would take me a long time to realize that his delusions weren't influenced by everything. Trying to insulate his environment to keep out things that might prick up suspicion is not only impossible but also pointless. The *evidence* a schizophrenic gives to support a delusion could be anything, things you would never imagine. For instance, if someone with schizophrenia believes there are listening devices planted around their room, your first question might be, "Well, who do you think would want to listen in on you?"

The patient may not be able to put his finger on who or what is targeting him, but he feels so strongly that it is happening that he cannot be dissuaded. Instead he may point to evidence. One day, someone could be changing a light fixture in his room. He might see the wires in the wall and say, "Aha! I told you so!"

During the summer of 2006, after months of little contact between Dad and Pat, I negotiated to have Pat come back to the office. I told Dad about the work I had been taking home with me and how Pat had helped with it. He said okay. I told Pat, and Pat said he'd come back to work on Monday morning. The lack of direct communication between the two was typical, perhaps even dysfunctional, and it didn't help matters, considering the recent amplification of Pat's symptoms.

Soon it was like nothing had ever happened. Neither of them ever spoke of Pat's six-month absence.

I was excited that going back to work meant that Pat would have to socialize more often. Having my own issues with social anxiety, I know that exposure to people is the only way to beat it back. If you have too much time by yourself, away from other people, especially never coming into contact with strangers, it's that much harder to face social situations without crippling anxiety. But going to work didn't make him want to do any more socializing. He missed out on several concerts that summer while his friends or I went to see his favorite bands. He would ask me to bring things home for him from a store, and I usually refused, hoping he'd face the music. Instead, he just went without.

Yet even at the office he was cold and detached. Uncle Larry, always the office comedian, started referring to Pat as Spock, after the unemotional, ingenious, ever-pragmatic Vulcan from *Star Trek*.

In autumn, I was taking an abnormal psychology class to fulfill my minor in psychology. Abnormal psychology covers abnormalities in behavior considered markedly outside the realm of what is acceptable within a person's culture. We studied psychopathology and every diagnosis in the *Diagnostic and Statistical Manual* (*DSM*), the holy grail for mental health practitioners. Very early on we discussed schizophrenia. My best friend Hannah was sitting next to me, and she leaned over as we took notes. "Sarah, doesn't that sound like Pat?" She asked this almost in jest, but I detected a little bit of anxiety in her voice.

"Of course not," I answered immediately. My perception of schizophrenia was of a stark-raving lunatic. And Pat didn't have hallucinations. He wasn't dangerous. But I had to shake off the stereotypes. In class students were realizing that there is no cut-and-dried definition of mental illness, just a list of criteria and a broad spectrum of how symptoms could be expressed. And students are often warned not to start diagnosing people, as many "symptoms" taken separately can be conceived of as being very normal parts of a person's personality. Clusters of symptoms only become pathological in some people. Hannah touched my arm, hoping she hadn't offended me.

I looked down at my notes: "delusions, social withdrawal, thought disorder, unemotional, flat affect, reduced ability to plan and execute activity, memory problems, loss of interest in former hobbies, and poor self-care (hygiene)."

"No, no. He's not this bad," I whispered to her. I told myself a schizophrenic wouldn't still be working every day, playing guitar and recording songs, and just generally taking care of himself. As I studied for my midterm, I felt completely certain he couldn't be schizophrenic. The diagnostic criteria seemed so obvious, and Pat's issues were so obscure.

He stopped talking outdoors again. In the evening when I got home, I would find the vent in the master bathroom on, rattling away. He offered no explanation for it. Then I found that the bathroom door had a huge crack in it. It was up high, about where a fist would go. Pat said he'd been drunk and didn't know how it happened. I became so concerned about his drinking, I often left parties and other gatherings early, thinking that at home I could at least keep an eye on him.

Finishing my last year in college, there were a lot of decisions to face. I didn't mind working in the family business. It suited me fine, but I was sure it was time for me to get out of New Orleans for a while. I thought about other states, other schools, places I hadn't considered while I was applying to undergraduate schools because money was so limited and I was afraid of taking out student loans. I was ready to see new things, new people, something completely different. Part of me wanted to go as far away as I could, to do graduate study in England or Scotland. Another part of me was scared to death to go out on my own. And what about Pat? I never imagined being so far from him I couldn't see him whenever I wanted.

To complicate things further, I started dating Gavin, and we were getting serious. He had just finished his degree in communications and was always talking about moving to New York City. We held off talking about where all this would lead us, but we both knew we'd be staying together.

Introducing Gavin to Pat was intimidating. If Pat was feeling himself, he'd certainly like him. They listened to the same music and liked the same films.

We were very similar, so of course he had a lot in common with Pat too. But Pat had been so quirky lately. I wasn't worried that something odd would scare Gavin away; rather, I was afraid he wouldn't get to know the real Pat. It would hurt my feelings if Gavin thought my brother was creepy, someone who made him uncomfortable. I conveyed to Gavin how important Pat is to me, and he was determined to be his friend. He stayed at our house for much of my last semester in college.

With a social grace unheard of in my family, Gavin was always warm, friendly, and even accommodating with my relatives. They said Gavin was always wide-eyed and smiling, but I suspect he was just trying to muscle through the awkwardness. Little did I know he'd have a front-row seat for Pat's complete and utter unraveling.

Convinced that his behavior was adding up to something significant, I called his old psychologist Dr. Milner to talk to him about it. "He's fine, Sarah. I saw him just last month."

"He came to see you?" I was stunned.

"Yes, he was worried about something." He began to divulge privileged information, but it wasn't anything I hadn't already heard. "Pat came in and said he felt like people were watching him, following him. He thought strangers knew who he was. I assured him this wasn't true. We went for a ride over to the Piggly Wiggly and walked around together. I showed him that no one knew him and no one was spying."

"And he accepted that?" I asked.

"Oh, he knows it's true," he said in his jovial way.

"See, I don't think he does," I said.

"Sarah, I promise you, he's just acting out. Aren't you about to leave for graduate school?"

"I've been talking about going out of state."

"Well, I think that's great. Pat told me a little about it, and it's my opinion he's just acting out because he doesn't want you to go."

"He doesn't want me to go?"

"Just like he was upset when you moved away after high school. Now you're going even further away, and he doesn't know how to handle it."

"Did he say this to you?"

"No, but you have to read between the lines," he said.

"But doctor, he's never done anything like this before."

"He's never been faced with these circumstances before."

"Is that what his psychiatrist thinks, too?"

"I can give you the number for Dr. Hollis, if you'd like to talk to him too."

I left multiple messages for Hollis and never heard back. I assumed he thought I was prying into his therapy, but I had no desire to know what he talked about in session. I needed someone to tell me he was okay. I saw Pat as a train going off the tracks, and no one wanted to help me stop it.

Nothing Dr. Milner said set me at ease. I didn't believe that Pat would act out. He had always been so blunt and forthcoming with his feelings. Furthermore, I took offense at the assumption he would be so out of sorts at the mere thought of me leaving. My brother always loved me, but he was never possessive of me. Besides, in the last year, he had been acting so strangely that he didn't seem very concerned about anything I did.

A week later, while Gavin and I were falling asleep in bed, there was a knock on my door. Gavin woke up and asked me if I'd heard it. In a daze, I went to the door and opened it. Pat was standing there holding a remote control.

"What?" I was confused.

"Tell me who put the listening devices in the remote."

"Pat, what?" I was getting angry.

"I know you know who did it. Somebody had to let them into the house. Just tell me who they are."

I was at the end of my rope, "Pat, go to bed. Leave me alone. I have to be up in the morning." I started to close the door, and he pushed it open with his hand. "Stop it, Pat! Cut the crap and go to bed!" I slammed the door and locked it.

"I'm sorry," I told Gavin.

"It's okay. I'm sorry, too."

"I just can't take it anymore."

The next morning while Gavin slept, I went to class. Afterward, I found that Pat wasn't at the office. I went about my usual routine until my dad called me into his office. As I walked down the hall, I passed Uncle Larry. He looked as white as a sheet.

Dad gestured for me to sit down. "I had to send Pat home."

"What's going on?" The air suddenly felt thick. I couldn't sit.

"Larry told me Pat was convinced that Clint Herbert," a coworker and the only other male close to Pat's age in the office, "was stalking him."

"Stalking?" Clint was new. I couldn't even recall a time when he said more than two words to Pat.

"He swore to Larry that Clint was rifling through his mail, checking his phone messages and his e-mails. He said he could *prove* it."

It was inconceivable. "Why would Clint do that?"

"There is no reason. No one would do that. It's—"

"It's crazy."

Dad shut his eyes and continued. "I had to send him home. I was afraid he would make a scene."

"Does Clint know?"

"God, no. And I don't want anyone to tell him."

"I told you he was telling me things like this, things that didn't make any sense." My eyes began to well up.

"I know," he sighed. Dad is always able to find composure even when it has been completely sucked out of a room. "I just didn't want to believe it was this bad. I thought it was a misunderstanding or a passing phase."

"I left messages for Dr. Hollis, but he doesn't return my calls."

"Give me the number. Your mother and I will get in touch with him."

"Can I go home? Gavin is there, and if Pat's there—" I was finally scared that Pat would frighten Gavin away.

"Go ahead." His eyes were searching his desk, trying to think of the magic antidote for this situation. Nothing would come.

I gave him the number, doubting he'd hear from the elusive Dr. Hollis either. I gathered my things hurriedly. I didn't want to speak to anyone else at the office, not even Uncle Larry. The secret was out. Other people were involved now. It should have felt like I was getting somewhere, but it didn't. I felt judged. I felt protective of my brother. Not only did I want to scream at everyone for not intervening sooner, I wanted them to feel the sadness that was swallowing me up like kudzu vines choking an old house. It was impossible to know the right thing to do or what the future would hold. I guess that's why I've so often thought of schizophrenia as a fog.

When I reached the house, Pat was outside smoking. I found Gavin in my bedroom with a smile on his face.

"Everything okay?"

"Yeah, why?" he asked, putting down his book.

"Dad sent Pat home today." I explained to him the new delusions about our coworker. "Who knows how long he's felt that way."

"He did come in here at one point."

"He did?"

"He just stood in the doorway and asked me a question. He asked, 'What would you do if you thought people were watching you?'"

"What did you say?"

"I said, 'I would want to know why.' He nodded, and then he went out."

My stomach sank. I hoped he would try to convince Pat that no one was watching him. Pat seemed to have respect for Gavin; maybe he could appeal to reason. But reason wasn't going to make an appearance now. Pat felt so strongly that his suspicions were accurate that he had no interest in explanations otherwise.

Pat stayed home from work, and our parents took turns sleeping over to "keep an eye on him." Gavin flew to New York City to look for an apartment there. I began applying to graduate schools, but in the midst of Pat's problems, I failed to keep an appointment with my independent study mentor. It was almost Thanksgiving, and nothing seemed to be turning out as planned.

I came home from studying one evening to find Dad in the kitchen talking to Pat. They discussed his delusions for hours. Dad was trying to convince him that he wasn't being surveilled.

Suddenly Pat said, "Dad, I know."

"You know?" Dad was surprised.

"I know everything you're going to say even before you say it."

"What do you mean?"

"I can hear what you're going to say in my head before you actually speak."

"That's impossible, Pat."

"See? I knew you would say that!" He seemed to marvel at this newfound ability. He looked almost as scared as us. "Somebody must have put something in my head. If I'm in your head, someone could be in mine, listening to my thoughts."

In schizophrenia this symptom is called thought broadcasting. It is the belief that someone has access to your thoughts, as if they are being broadcast. It is a *positive symptom* because it is a departure from normal function, added by the illness rather than taken away. It has been suggested that thought broadcasting distinguishes schizophrenia from all other mental illness. It ties into other symptoms like thought insertion, in which patients believe their thoughts are not their own, and thought extraction, in which patients believe their thoughts are missing because they have been taken out of their mind. The overall idea is that they feel they have no control over their thoughts, but someone or something else does.

Years later in cognitive neuroscience, my professor, a neurologist himself, would offer a hypothesis for auditory hallucinations and thought broadcasting in schizophrenia. When a person tells you a phone number or street address and you keep it in mind while you find a pen to write it down, you're holding that information in short-term memory. You have to get the pen quickly because this kind of memory decays rapidly. In your mind it's as if you can still hear what has just been said. Psychologists Alan Baddeley and Graham Hitch called this the phonological loop of working memory. You use this working memory in order to take notes during a meeting or lecture. It contains auditory traces of what you've just heard and an articulatory loop that replays it. It's a kind of inner voice on a loop trying to hold on to the auditory information before it's forgotten entirely. The thing is that you know the inner voice is under your control; it's a part of your mind. It is suggested that in schizophrenia, patients do not recognize this inner voice as their own thoughts. They find it is completely alien, not under their control. It's no wonder that Pat would feel frightened and persecuted.

When I went to bed that night, Dad and Pat were still talking in the kitchen. Endless nights like these left the whole family exhausted. Communicating was supposed to solve problems, but here it did nothing other than ramp up anxiety and even resentment.

Out of the blue, I began having nightmares. In them I was usually looking for Pat with a feeling of dread. I remember one dream clearly. Someone had broken into the house, men dressed all in black with big guns. I thought they were people Pat owed money to, probably drug dealers. Before they could find me, I snuck to Pat's room. He wasn't there. I crept into the closet to hide, and inside it were these white trash bags. Touching one to see what was inside, I found Pat's head. It was the first time I ever woke up screaming.

In early December 2006, the psychiatrist finally met with Mom, Dad, and Pat. He spoke with them first one by one and then as a group. Dr. Hollis diagnosed Pat with paranoid schizophrenia. He found it particularly alarming to learn that in the past six or seven years Pat had gone from being an outgoing extrovert to a socially anxious introvert. I thought it was crazy he had been treating and medicating Pat for two years without gleaning this fact himself.

Pat was given a new, second-generation antipsychotic. Mom gave him the pills and watched him take them. Within a week he was taking them on his own and showed vast improvement. He stopped talking about delusions, started sleeping at night, and returned to work before Christmas. He didn't complain of any side effects, although he often had trouble getting out of bed.

For our last study meeting, I met my mentor, Professor Long, at a coffee shop close to my house. I sat outside on a patio so I had an excuse to wear sunglasses. Still, my puffy nose betrayed me.

"So what's been going on with you? You haven't been sick this whole time."

"Things have been complicated. It's my family. I live with my older brother and he's been sick lately."

"Sick?" He stirred his coffee.

I worked to clear the lump in my throat. I really didn't want to talk about it. "He was just diagnosed, finally, with paranoid schizophrenia."

"Sarah?" He sat up straight in his chair. He looked like he wanted to take my hand but resisted. "Sarah, why didn't you tell me about this?"

"It all just recently came to a head really."

"You didn't tell me all this was going on at home." He seemed visibly hurt. He proceeded to apologize to me. "I'm sorry if you felt like this was something you couldn't share with me. We've been meeting the whole semester. I wish you would have told me."

We didn't talk about existentialism in Romantic literature that day. We just talked about Pat, and then Professor Long went home. I had known the professor less than a year, but he wanted to comfort me. I didn't know how to let him. We had never talked about our personal lives before, other than perhaps where we were going on vacation. He didn't even know that I had a brother before that day. I didn't know how to open up to him all of a sudden, least of all about someone so close to my heart.

I got another coffee and sat on the patio smoking. I had been worried sick about Pat for a year, while friends kept reassuring me that it was probably nothing to worry about. Maybe I had been talking to the wrong people. Maybe I should have told my professor.

My boyfriend and a few close friends knew of the diagnosis. People didn't seem to really understand what schizophrenia is. There is so much more to the illness than simply doing things that might seem weird or irrational. What I have found is that there is a general misunderstanding about schizophrenia, that many people don't know there are different kinds and different degrees to which people display symptoms. There is a wide perception of the schizophrenic as being wild in his gesticulations, unkempt, irrational, talking to himself out loud, and even dangerous. And this may be true for some sufferers, but not all, and certainly not for Pat.

I took my finals in a daze. My abnormal psychology test felt like a cruel joke. I felt like I had lost my brother and no one around me understood. I wanted to shake everyone by the shoulders and say, "Don't you understand? Don't you see what we've lost?" Pat wasn't a weirdo. He wasn't a strange guy. He was a smart, funny, brilliant man who was now lost in a fog of paranoia. Even with medication, he'd never be the same.

11

Facing the Diagnosis

There is a strange comfort in finally getting a diagnosis. While Pat was losing his grip on reality, I felt like I was also losing mine. Now that we knew schizophrenia was the cause of his erratic behavior, all the other possibilities fell by the wayside. It wasn't drug use or alcoholism. It wasn't a dietary issue. The planets weren't oddly aligned, and a body snatcher hadn't replaced my brother with an alien. But with the diagnosis there comes the hard reality of the disease and the difficulty of treating it.

When I was learning about schizophrenia in school, I thought I grasped the signs, the symptoms, and the prognosis. Instead, I had only glimpsed a handful of notable symptoms and heard maybe one case-study example. More than anything, what I took away was a great deal of relief that I had never known the raw fearsomeness that schizophrenia presented. My psychology minor—*minor* was a very apt word—couldn't prepare me for the hurdles ahead.

Schizophrenia certainly isn't an obvious illness. The onset can be any combination of behavioral changes, including positive and negative symptoms. There are two kinds of onset: acute and insidious. Acute onset happens rapidly, and diagnosis often occurs in the emergency room. These cases are easier to treat, likely because the changes in behavior are sudden and easily noticed. Yesterday the patient was fine, and today he's convinced aliens have put listening devices in his fillings. An insidious onset, like Pat's, creeps up at a snail's pace. Changes occur in such small increments that they can almost

Table 11.1.   DSM-IV Criteria for Schizophrenia

1. Characteristic symptoms: Two* or more of the following most of the time during a period of one month.
   - A. Delusions
   - B. Hallucinations
   - C. Disorganized speech (such as confused, repetitive speech or jumping quickly from topic to topic)
   - D. Grossly disorganized behavior (e.g., confronting others without logical reason) or catatonic behavior (e.g., rigid muscles or lack of response to the environment)
   - E. Negative symptoms (e.g., lack of emotion, social withdrawal, neglect of personal hygiene)
   * Only one of these symptoms is required if:
     1. Hallucinations include a voice making continuous commentary on the person's thoughts.
     2. Hallucinations include two or more voices conversing with each other.
     3. Delusions are *bizarre* (e.g., thought broadcasting).
2. The person has experienced a marked decrease in their ability to function socially or occupationally.
3. The disturbance has persisted for at least six months (including one month of symptoms mentioned above).
4. The person is not experiencing extreme mood episodes associated with schizoaffective disorder or mood disorder or these mood episodes have been brief.
5. The symptoms do not suggest any developmental disorder such as autism or mental retardation.

always be explained away. "Oh, he's just sleepy. He had a rough week. He wants to be left alone." If you see only one or two of these symptoms at any one time, you would never jump to the conclusion of incurable mental illness. Table 11.1 outlines the criteria for being diagnosed with schizophrenia.

I have seen shades of these symptoms (see table 11.2) in my own behavior; perhaps many people do. There are any number of reasons that a person would stop hanging around their circle of friends. Social isolation, keeping just to one's own immediate family, doesn't necessarily send up red flags. Many introverts spend a number of days at a time alone. Everyone is guilty of procrastinating and putting off important tasks. A whole spectrum of anxious behavior includes ruminating on past disappointments, failures, or mishaps. Many people drink and smoke cigarettes with reckless abandon without having schizophrenia. Pat did not seem stressed out. He was never unkempt, and he did not seem unable to cope with minor complications. He was stubborn, but far more than 1 percent of the population is stubborn. He didn't talk to himself and never has.

Furthermore, each one of these symptoms fits into a broad array of psychological diagnoses. Perhaps a psychiatrist or psychologist with years of

Table 11.2.   Sample of Early Warning Signs of Schizophrenia

- Bizarre behavior
- Sleep problems (oversleeping or difficulty sleeping)
- Dropping out of life activities
- Social isolation
- Neglecting self-care (e.g., hygiene, clothing)
- Ruminating on past events (often negative events)
- Deterioration of work or school performance
- Drug or alcohol abuse
- Rigid stubbornness
- Mood problems (e.g., anxiety, depression, sudden irritability)
- Lack of emotion
- Inability to derive pleasure (even if doing things that once brought pleasure)
- Feeling apathetic toward big life events
- Hypersensitivity to criticism
- Lack of motivation or goal-oriented behaviors
- Inappropriate response (e.g., laughing at something sad)
- Unusual gait
- Clumsy motor skills
- Unusual posture or gestures
- Involuntary movements of the tongue or mouth
- Poor memory and concentration
- Difficulty interpreting social cues
- Obsessive compulsive tendencies
- Racing thoughts
- Difficulty expressing thoughts or not having much to say (also called poverty of speech or alogia)

experience would see schizophrenia as clear as day, but a person who knows Pat even just a little bit would have their perspective tangled up in the past, envisioning the person he used to be. For those who knew him before the onset, there is a deep disparity between who he was then and who he is now. The things he was interested in and the way his life was headed are no longer a reality after the psychotic break. I had never considered that mental illness could appear seemingly out of nowhere.

Diagnosis wasn't the end. There were steps to be taken. The first thing Dr. Hollis addressed was medication. He explained to us that it might take a while to find the right kind of antipsychotic and dosage. *Antipsychotic.* I knew that word. It stuck in my throat. It sounded like a kind of armor, something that could be machine-gunned without so much as a dent. "So this is what they're for. I guess that makes sense," I thought. "There's no way I can tell people he's on antipsychotics without them thinking—" I checked myself. This wasn't the time to be thinking about myself or how I felt.

What Dr. Hollis didn't tell us was that 15 percent of people diagnosed with schizophrenia only respond moderately to medication, while another 15 percent don't respond at all.[1]

Antipsychotics work by blocking dopamine receptors in the brain. By doing so they decrease the positive symptoms associated with schizophrenia. Dopamine is a neurotransmitter, a chemical used by nerve cells to help them communicate with other nerve cells. In the brain, it plays a large role in cognition, mood, attention, sleep (remember, Pat also sleepwalks and sleep-eats), voluntary movement, memory, and motivation. It powers the reward system of the brain, giving the sensation of pleasure when something is accomplished and providing motivation.

In schizophrenia there is inexplicable dopamine dysfunction in the brain. There is decreased dopamine in the prefrontal cortex, which moderates attention and planning, and an increased amount of dopamine in the mesolimbic pathway, often referred to as the reward pathway. The reward center of the brain is powered by dopamine. This area is thought to help us set goals, anticipate rewards, and feel pleasure when the goal is met. Here we can see how symptoms like lack of emotion, low motivation, social withdrawal, loss of pleasure in old activities, and decreased ability to function socially and occupationally crop up in schizophrenia. I had a teacher suggest that the prefrontal cortex is ultimately responsible for so much decision making and behavior inhibition that it is the seat of personality. Dopaminergic dysfunction is also associated with autism, attention deficit hyperactivity disorder, Parkinson's disease, and drug abuse.

The problem with antipsychotics is that they address dopamine dysfunction without treating the cause of the dysfunction. Science has yet to reveal what causes these changes in the brain. The medication has many serious side effects. An MD once described antipsychotics to me as "blindly throwing a bag of knives at a target in the dark."

"We don't know what causes it," he said. "All we can do is hope that the drugs do more good than harm."

You've probably heard of antipsychotics developed in the 1950s referred to as "typical" or "first-generation" antipsychotics. Some commonly prescribed examples include Thorazine (chlorpromazine) and Haldol (haloperidol). By 1964, a new movement disorder was classified as a result of taking these medications. Tardive dyskinesia (TD) is characterized by uncontrollable movements of the limbs, smacking of the lips, facial grimacing, swaying, puffing of the cheeks, or repetitive movements of the tongue, mouth, or jaw. Other side effects from antipsychotics include sedation, tremors, rigid muscles, blurred vision, and skin rashes.

Atypical, "second-generation" antipsychotics were developed later, their difference being that they cause fewer extrapyramidal motor control problems. Fewer people get TD if they take atypicals, but some still develop the disorder. The elimination of adverse effects on motor control improves functioning and hopefully leads to better medication compliance.[2] Although many claim to have fewer side effects than with first-generation drugs, second-generation antipsychotics are associated with weight gain,[3] development of type 2 diabetes,[4] and high cholesterol.[5] Over time, many have argued that the two generations of medicine turned out to be too similar to differentiate.

Dr. Hollis didn't describe integral aspects of the illness to my parents or my brother. Perhaps he sensed that they were too befuddled by the diagnosis to remember anything else he would have said. He never mentioned that antipsychotics do not treat the negative or cognitive symptoms of schizophrenia. So while we are tranquilizing the positive symptoms that cause so much anxiety and distress, many other functions are still impaired, functions necessary for independent living. For a list of the positive, cognitive, and negative symptoms, see table 11.3.

Pat was given just one medication (an atypical antipsychotic), and we mistook that as par for the course. My family didn't realize that schizophrenia patients often take a wide variety of drugs, a cocktail of multiple antipsychotic, antianxiety, and antidepressant medications. The road ahead would have many bumps and curves. Pat seemed to take the prescription seriously and was diligent in taking the medication, although he never said anything about the diagnosis.

Table 11.3. Symptoms of Schizophrenia

Positive Symptoms	Cognitive Symptoms	Negative Symptoms
Hallucinations	Difficulty focusing	Apathy
Delusions	Poor working memory	Social withdrawal
Movement disorder	Difficulty with planning	Flat affect (facial expression)
Thought disorder	and decision making	Low motivation
(e.g., word salad)		Poor self-care (personal hygiene)
		Anhedonia (inability to experience pleasure)
		Alogia (poverty of speech)
		Anosognosia (lack of self-awareness)

Table 11.4.   Phases of Schizophrenia

Phase 1: Prodrome	Phase 2: Active	Phase 3: Residual	Phase 4: Relapse or Recovery

Characterized by:
  Social withdrawal
  Anxiety
  Poor attention
  Unusual thoughts
	Characterized by:
	  Delusions
	  Hallucinations
		Characterized by:
		  Predominantly
		  negative
		  symptoms
			Recovery or relapse
			  into the active phase

Dr. Hollis was hopeful that Pat would be responsive to an antipsychotic because it was the very beginning of his illness. Because I was not consulted during the diagnosis, Hollis considered the recent delusion about his coworker spying on him to be Pat's first episode. No one mentioned the year prior, when Pat accused Dad and the roofers of conspiring against him. Why is this important? Because schizophrenia follows a cycle, and each time the patient goes through the cycle the likelihood of their recovery decreases (see table 11.4).

What is recovery in schizophrenia? It doesn't mean that all the symptoms of schizophrenia are gone, but rather that they are managed. Patients don't lapse back into active-phase symptoms like delusions or hallucinations; they work through negative symptoms, and they are able to recover their social and occupational lives again. Recovery in schizophrenia looks like normal life but requires hard work, therapy, and support. There is no "full recovery." Something stressed to us from the very beginning was that nothing was going to give Pat back to us whole. He could live a normal life, but probably never the life he was leading before, or the life we thought he would lead. Coming to terms with that, however, took much longer.

A monumental obstacle that stands in the way of recovery and leads more often to relapse is anosognosia, a lack of awareness of self and one's illness. Many people diagnosed with severe mental illness do not recognize that they are afflicted. From the beginning it was very important for me to hear Pat talk about his diagnosis. I wanted him to affirm or question it. He never spoke of it, and I was too afraid to bring it up. Our parents also had the attitude of letting sleeping dogs lie. As long as Pat was taking his medication, no one was willing to push his buttons. We were all so exhausted by his active-phase symptoms that we couldn't dare face them again. Trying to talk a person out of a delusion feels like some kind of oblique torture, testing your own faculties until you feel your own grip on reality slide away from you.

We hoped that as long as he stayed on the medication the delusions would not come back, but there are "flare-ups" that can arise and that eventually lead to getting off medication. If Pat felt a little paranoid, he could decide the medication was somehow hurting him instead of helping him—for instance, keeping him from being vigilant or seeing something important. Without support, he could go off medication and suffer a full-fledged relapse into florid psychosis.

Books on schizophrenia tried to address this issue. Most suggested a tight support network—not just the family, but his mental health providers as well. They stressed the importance of therapy, not just seeing a psychiatrist on a monthly basis, which Pat agreed to, but also seeing a psychologist on a weekly basis, and hopefully getting into group therapy with other people diagnosed with schizophrenia. Pat scoffed at these ideas. Without my parents' help, there was no convincing him.

There are many things you have to learn about schizophrenia as you go. The things you don't know are the things you'd never think to ask until it's staring you in the face.

A person who is mentally healthy at age twenty-one is always going to be healthy, right? Wrong. The average onset of schizophrenia in males is between the ages of sixteen and twenty-five, and between twenty-five and thirty in women.[6] Pat was twenty-three when his strange behavior began. The majority of those with onset after age thirty are women, while onset after forty is very rare. Imagine a person you knew in high school or college but have seen little of since. Now imagine they have been diagnosed with schizophrenia since you last saw them. What does that look like? Are you only imagining the *weird* students you knew? Let's be fair—if being strange was an indicator of severe mental illness, we'd be getting help for these people long before the onset of their illness. We might even know how to prevent onset. No, weirdness is not in the diagnostic criteria for schizophrenia. Just imagine anyone you haven't seen in a while between the ages of eighteen and thirty-five. Now imagine they've been diagnosed with schizophrenia. You might have conjured up images of straitjackets, sterile corridors, padded rooms, and beds with straps.

Film and television gave me the impression that people with schizophrenia spend their lives in mental hospitals. I know full well that the nation was deinstitutionalized, but for some reason, schizophrenia seemed like an illness that required hospitalization, like cancer or AIDS. I didn't think that as soon as he was diagnosed the doctor would have him sent away to a mental hospital, but I imagined if his frightening delusions returned, we would have a place to turn. He would go somewhere where doctors knew how to stop all his symptoms.

Dr. Milner, his former psychologist, told me this was not the case. He said that if Pat was ever getting too agitated to handle, I had to call the police. I would have to tell the officer that Pat has schizophrenia and then make a convincing argument that Pat is a danger to himself or to others. He would be taken to the hospital and treated, but without his consent they could not keep him there for longer than a week. "I'm not sure—probably a couple of days to a week."

"A week? What good is that?" I asked.

"It's the law. It's the longest they can hold him against his will."

"If the police come, is he arrested? Are they going to handcuff him and put him in the back of the car?"

"They would probably handcuff him and put him in the back of a squad car. They don't book him; he's not under arrest."

"I don't know what's scarier, calling the police or letting him accuse our neighbors and coworkers of spying on him."

"If there's a pattern of violence, you'll likely establish a relationship with law enforcement, and the next time they come out they won't need you to answer so many questions. They'll know what you're dealing with," he said.

"Great, I can't wait to establish rapport with the cops dragging my brother away." My eyes were filled with tears when I hung up the phone.

The outlook for schizophrenia is pessimistic: They seldom stay on medication. They have flare-ups of positive symptoms. There were many more negative symptoms we could look forward to. We had to be vigilant. How does one stay vigilant against an illness another person has?

I wanted to stay proactive and face down the diagnosis. I tried to read books and learn about the illness faster than it could take over Pat's mind. I suppose I've always been a fixer. I can't stand an unsolvable puzzle. I will devote all my time to getting the conundrum off my plate. But schizophrenia can't be solved. It is unpredictable and impossible to nail down. Somewhere deep down I knew there were other feelings I had to sort out, feelings I had to feel in order to move forward, like grief. Who had time for grief?

Learning more about schizophrenia can mean learning just how helpless you and your loved one are. The best books and documentaries that I uncovered were ones that addressed coping. Feeling grief, guilt, and even resentment are normal after the diagnosis. Finding ways to cope with those feelings is vital to your own health.

While I was trying to sort out a plan of action, our parents were still trying to wrap their heads around what had happened. I looked to the future while they took a hard look at the past. More than anything, they wanted to know, why Pat?

Schizophrenia does run in families. A person is more likely to develop the illness if they have a relative with the disease. While it only occurs in just 1 percent of the general population, it occurs in 10 percent of people who have first-degree relatives with schizophrenia.[7] Children of parents who both have schizophrenia are about 40 percent more likely to develop the disease. If an individual diagnosed has an identical twin, the risk of that twin developing the disease is 28 percent. Genes confer the same risk of schizophrenia in children whether they are adopted or not.[8]

While these data suggest a strong genetic component to schizophrenia, scientists have not found any one gene solely responsible for its development. This leads to the assumption that it is a combination of nature and nurture that leads to schizophrenia. But the environmental factors uncovered are diverse and inconsistent. These encompass living further away from the equator, living in a colder climate, growing up in urban areas, prenatal exposure to toxoplasmosis or influenza or maternal stress, prenatal vitamin D deficiency, and obstetric complications.[9]

Despite the fact that these factors are common enough to be linked to schizophrenia, they don't apply to everyone. No one else in our family has schizophrenia. There has been no other mental illness diagnosed in the family. Mom had no obstetric complications or infections during pregnancy. She wasn't aware of any unusual psychosocial stress or vitamin deficiency. We live near the equator and grew up in a rural area. Gene expression is an unpredictable dance of nature and nurture.

Still, we sifted through our back pages hoping to find a culprit. Maybe we just wanted someone or something to blame. My maternal grandmother had the most evidence to present. She mentioned her father who spent most of his adult life in a VA hospital. But he developed posttraumatic stress disorder after serving in World War I. What about her aunt who committed suicide? If a woman kills herself at age nineteen after being spurned by a lover, it doesn't necessarily mean she suffered from schizophrenia. My grandmother had a cousin who committed suicide as well. "He was never right in the head," she said. For all we know, there could be virtually any reason he killed himself, though schizophrenia cannot be ruled out.

On Dad's side of the family, there was no suicide, but there was an array of anxiety. Anxiety was something we women used to say ran in the family. But none of these histories could have warned us of what was in store for Pat.

Research also links schizophrenia to childhood trauma, including physical abuse, sexual abuse, the death of a parent, neglect, emotional or psychosocial abuse, and bullying. A recent study found that schizophrenia patients were 2.72 times more likely to report experiencing trauma in childhood.[10] As far as I knew, Pat hadn't experienced anything like that, but I had to be sure. For my own peace of mind, I couldn't just assume. When I asked Pat if he recalled any childhood trauma, he said no.

"Well, were you ever bullied?" I asked. I stood in the kitchen watching him open a bottle of wine.

"No way. I'd never let someone bully me."

I knew he was probably right. He was always bigger than other kids. "What about getting spanked?"

He shrugged. "It was scary, especially if I didn't feel like I had done anything wrong, but I wouldn't call it traumatic."

"What do you consider traumatic?"

"You know, like a car accident, getting beat up or mugged. Nothing like that ever happened to me."

"Did you feel like you were at risk of that happening? When you went out with your friends, were you in dangerous neighborhoods?" I probed a little further.

"No, I wouldn't have gone somewhere dangerous." He looked at me quizzically for a moment, perhaps not understanding my line of questioning. "Do you feel like you were traumatized?"

I was taken aback and shook my head, not knowing how to answer. "I don't think so. I don't think my childhood was that much different from anyone else's."

"You know what's really traumatizing?" He didn't look at me as he spoke. "Not knowing who to trust," he said, picking up the television remote. I knew he didn't want to talk about it anymore. It's a subject I often think of revisiting with him, but when Pat's feeling well and we're having a good conversation about lighthearted things, I just don't want to spoil it. I leave exploring "trauma" to his therapist.

Smoking cannabis is known to increase the risk of developing schizophrenia, and the risk becomes greater the more cannabis is used.[11] Of course we all had to wonder if he would be healthy now had he never smoked weed or had he not smoked so much of it. But that idea is circular. I also have to wonder if the marijuana was a form of self-medication through the insidious onset of schizophrenia; many people struggling with mental illness use substances to mitigate symptoms. If I can't put my finger on the very beginning of the schizophrenia, the moment when there was no turning back, there's no way to say which came first, the drug use or the illness, or if they are related at all.

Mom, Dad, and I went into autopilot. There was grief for the young man we had lost and for the future he would likely not have, but it was on the back burner. We knew there was much we still had to learn about schizophrenia and Pat's treatment, but it all had to wait. Pat's fog was beginning to lift, and he wanted to return to full-time work. The rest of us were stunned and lost and unable to decide what to do next. Paralyzed by confusion and worry, we felt powerless at the same time that we wanted to help, to cure him somehow and set him back on the right path.

Mom and Dad were wounded. I imagined there would be some small comfort in going through this together, but they seemed isolated in their grief. Perhaps they blamed each other for Pat's illness, for not recognizing that something was wrong. It had to be hard to face the fact that environment could contribute to the illness. One could fill an ocean with all the things they could have done differently. As I said before, each of us is well versed in being too hard on ourselves. I know I struggled with seeing the illness as my fault. I knew he was smoking a lot of marijuana, but I knew so many other college students who did too.

I kept thinking I must have pushed him away. Pat always told me about his feelings. Why didn't he tell me when he felt like the world was growing sinister, out to get him? I was sure it had to be something I did wrong that curtailed our communication. But again, there was not enough time to sort through that pain and make sense of it. We were all holding our breath, waiting for the other shoe to drop. The only way to know if the medicine was working depended on what Pat told us, and I worried he would hide his delusions from us.

A month after the diagnosis, I was shopping with Dad, looking for luggage to take to New York. He was quiet, but I assumed he was just tired. I knew he was sad that I was moving away. The reality of not seeing me every day was almost too much for him to talk about. He tried to put on his most pragmatic air in helping me pack and plan. Leaving the store, we got into the car, but he didn't start it. He hung his head low, looking at his lap. I thought that Pat's situation and my moving away had broken him. When he finally spoke, he kept apologizing for disappointing me. I didn't understand. Then he explained that he and Mom were getting a divorce.

I was leaving for New York City in three weeks. I was starting graduate study there in the fall. All I could think about was the mess I was leaving behind.

Part 3

FALLOUT

12

Denial

Moving to New York City is a conundrum of emotional extremes. I felt either intense excitement or immense fear. Part of me couldn't believe where I was. I swooned in Central Park, on Broadway, at the Empire State Building, in Rockefeller Center. It's the most recognizable city in the world. Everywhere I looked, I saw a place where they filmed this movie or that TV show. I had visited before, but actually living there was impossible. How did I get here?

There were other realities that hit me like a ton of bricks. So many industries are housed in New York that career possibilities are endless. Straight out of my undergrad, I couldn't figure out where I fit in or what I wanted to do. The longer I dragged my feet the bigger the gap in my resume. Meanwhile the competition is cutthroat, and the resumes of other potential hires show a straight trajectory toward a particular area. Where does an English major go? One false move and I could end up banished to a certain area forever. I thought I could do anything, but employers didn't feel the same way. It was 2007, and there weren't many jobs out there to be had.

After the move, I quit smoking—not because of the money, but rather because it was frowned upon. It didn't seem like anyone in New York smoked anymore. Perhaps it was the freezing temperatures outside.

I was dazzled by snow. Then I realized it was so cold outside that the snow would stick around and turn to ice. I lived in Brooklyn for less than a week before I slipped on the ice. I was so embarrassed. How do people get to work and school in this weather?

Many things were suddenly too expensive. Eating out was impossible for us, and neither Gavin nor I knew how to cook anything that didn't come in a can. Getting around took longer than it did in New Orleans. I couldn't take cabs everywhere. I now had to wait for a subway train to get around. How does that factor into how and when I leave for work? And every line is different. Some are much more reliable than others.

The subways, at first glance, are a labyrinthine mess of express trains, shortened services, and expensive transit cards. Looking for an apartment and a job meant considering neighborhoods I had never heard of. Were they safe? Sometimes a very safe neighborhood would border a particularly unsafe one. I myself lived in Bedford-Stuyvesant, Brooklyn. The neighborhood was home to the Marcy Housing Projects. Rappers like Jay-Z and Lil' Kim grew up there. It was mostly residential, mostly African American, and still prey to a lot of crime. Some of our friends, even native New Yorkers, wouldn't come to visit our new apartment.

Nothing bad ever happened while we lived there, but walking to and from the subway station could be a harrowing experience for me. A teenage boy followed me for blocks once, yelling at my back over and over again, "Hey, white girl! Hey, white girl!" I got used to tuning things out, and the neighborhood got used to seeing my face.

While looking for a place, Gavin insisted we not be on the first floor. He didn't want to have the sidewalk right outside his window. "It freaks me out," he said.

I thought about it for a long time. "I guess it doesn't really matter to me."

"But people walk by right outside your window. When you're watching TV or sleeping, all that's separating you might be a pane of glass."

"But everyone is right outside every window here. You're surrounded by people all the time." You can see your neighbor from your second-floor window, even though they're three floors up, standing in their kitchen, making dinner. And if there's no building there, it's construction workers outside your window. There are always people here. My feelings about being "surrounded" should have clued me in at the time, but I skimmed right over them.

Living in a matchbook-size apartment, I really had to reevaluate my personal possessions. Keep only what you need. Would I ever have a normal kitchen, a car, a fireplace, a dog, or a walk-in closet?

The city was inhospitable. I had to wait in line to do anything. Asking someone for directions was usually seen as highly intrusive. People could be instantly rude and unfriendly. It seemed like there was a panhandler on every subway staircase. I started wearing headphones and listening to music everywhere I went. How will my grandmother visit me if she can't get up and down the subway stairs and most stations don't have elevators? Besides, I couldn't imagine my Maw-Maw who was born in a barn in Mississippi enjoying the hustling and bustling crowds. Did I isolate myself by moving here? New York was beginning to feel like a mistake.

Without friends around to see me through, the bad seemed to outweigh the good. Every day felt like a struggle. I often found myself regaling people with stories of New Orleans. After Katrina, I thought it was unsafe to love a city so strongly when it could be ripped away from me by a single hurricane. After I moved away, all I could think about were the comforts of home. Family and friends weren't going to stop by. I couldn't laze around on the porch on a Sunday afternoon. I couldn't go to the grocery store and buy live crabs or fresh andouille. Oysters cost twice as much.

I traded the stress I left in Louisiana for a whole new kind of stress: life in the metropolis. And I was no ordinary southerner transplanted to Brooklyn. I was an introverted southerner with severe social anxiety, the breadth of which I could not appreciate until I was taken entirely away from the place I had known my whole life.

I was in the subway the first time it happened. I was standing on the platform with Gavin. A large group of teenagers nearby had just gotten out of school. Suddenly I felt flushed and nauseous. Gavin was speaking to me, but the sound was changing. My hearing grew tinny. My heart raced, and I was burning up. I didn't understand what was happening to me. He saw the blood draining from my face and grabbed my arm.

"Do you need to sit down?"

"Yes," I said at first. It was twenty degrees outside, but sweat was pouring down my back. "Wait, no. No, we have to get out of here."

"What?"

It was getting hard to speak. I thought I would lose consciousness. "We have to get out of the subway. I can't be down here, underground."

I lumbered up the subway steps slowly. Once outside, my light-headedness lifted. My body felt terribly weak, like I had just finished a marathon.

"What happened down there?" Gavin asked.

"I don't know. I suddenly felt like I would keel over," I said quietly, hoping nobody else would hear.

"Are you hungry?"

"No, I ate. I don't know what it was. I felt totally out of control."

"Has this happened before?"

"Maybe. The only thing I can compare it to is taking a pain pill on an empty stomach. Do you know what I mean? How did you feel when you had your wisdom teeth out and they sent you home with painkillers?"

"I just slept for days."

"Well, the painkillers made me light-headed and sick. My blood pressure would drop and I'd throw them up. It was miserable."

"Did you take something this morning?"

"No, I didn't. That's why I don't understand this."

"Maybe you just got too hot," he suggested, although it was unlikely.

"I don't know what happened first, if I got hot or sick."

I pulled my gloves and hat back on, finally feeling the chill. I was ready to brave the subway again. As we descended the stairs, the station took on an ominous aura for me. It was now a thing to be afraid of, something scary. In Louisiana, we don't have basements. Even graves are above ground. The smell in the subway reminded me of a mausoleum. The greasy cement was an old tomb. From then on, going down into the subway was a shaky experience. Would I get sick again? Are there fumes down here or something? What if I get sick and hot and can't get out?

The feeling hit me a few more times, sometimes on the subway train itself. If I could sit down, it would stave off my faintness. One afternoon, leaving the subway, I walked straight to a garbage can and threw up.

"Do you think maybe you have a problem with confined spaces?" Gavin was trying to be very sensitive with his inquiry.

"I never really thought about it," I said honestly.

"Well, how do you feel about rooms without windows?"

I shrugged. "I don't care."

"What about basements? Maybe it's an underground thing."

"I never went in a basement. They don't have real basements at home." Some homes have their front door on the second floor and refer to their first floor as the "basement."

"What about caves? Did you ever go into a cave?"

"There aren't any caves in New Orleans. Besides, how many people have gone into caves?"

"Where I grew up caves were a tourist attraction. Guides would give you a tour. Kids went there on field trips."

"Really? I don't think I'd have any interest in that." I thought about descending into a cave, and a cold chill ran up my spine. "No, I wouldn't like that at all."

"Even if there are plenty of other people there?"

"God, no. That's even worse."

"Why?"

"Because it's harder to get out."

He chuckled. "You wouldn't feel safer because other people are there with you?"

"No way. If anything, they make it worse. Other people are unpredictable."

"So you don't like it underground?"

"I guess so. It just feels unnatural to me. But then again I don't know if that's how I felt before I started getting dizzy spells in the subway. I wasn't aware of thinking anything in particular." I considered it for a while and said, "You know, there was one time last summer. I went to lunch with all the girls in the office. I had to sit in the very back of Mary's SUV. I thought I was going to go crazy."

"But then you weren't underground. There's something to that, Sarah."

"It was really hot outside. I felt faint and it bothered me that I couldn't just open a door and get out as soon as I wanted to. But that's weird, though. I used to ride in the back of cars all the time, two-door coupes where I didn't have a door. I rode in the back of my mom's car every day after school."

"In the subway, did you start thinking about how you couldn't get out? Is that when you started feeling bad?"

"No. No, I think I felt scared first. Then I had to get out."

"Scared of what?"

"Honestly, Gavin, I have no idea. Now when it happens, I'm just scared I'm going to pass out in front of everyone. I don't want to wake up on the floor of the train."

Visiting New Orleans was bittersweet. Part of me never wanted to go back to New York, and the other half was proud when everyone kept referring to me as a New Yorker. Gavin wanted to live in New York City forever, and I didn't want to let on how much that scared me.

Two months after the move, we went back to visit, staying in Pat's spare room. He had moved a few things around in the house, turning my old room into an office and music room. I took it as a good sign that he was evolving, personalizing his space, and making it more representative of his own style. He bought new artwork for the walls. Over the mantel in the living room was a large acrylic reproduction of Raphael's *The School of Athens.* My old house was now the philosopher's refuge.

He seemed perfectly well. He was working, taking care of himself, and not drinking every day. There was no delusional talk, no shiftiness or hesitation. He was talkative and enjoyed showing us his new things. We picked up where we left off. He played some new music for me and burned me some copies. For my birthday he had sent me an espresso machine, and we talked about how it works. It was the last present my brother ever bought for me.

When we invited him to go out with us that night, he wasn't interested. He was happy to stay home with his new video game console. Before, I had always had a sense of sorrow when I left him at home. We would be having a good conversation, enjoying our time together, but any attempt to leave the house and take it on the road was a barrier. I felt like I was shutting down the fun, taking away his good time. But if I let Pat have it his way, I never would have been able to go anywhere. He never seemed sad, but he didn't seem happy to see me go either.

Our parents were now living separately, but oddly enough they were spending a lot of time together. Mom said Dad was over at her house nearly every weekend doing work around the yard or house. She didn't let on, but I worried that this would send her mixed signals about where they stood. They had once been very close confidants, and Dad probably wasn't ready to lose that close connection. I thought he was jumping through hoops because he couldn't stand not being liked.

I sent my mom some books on schizophrenia, and I was excited to finally sit down and talk with her about them. Surprisingly, she hadn't looked at any of them yet. What's more, Pat's treatments had not changed at all since I had moved away four months earlier. He was still seeing Dr. Hollis once a month to talk about how the medication made him feel, but no one was treating him for his social anxiety or paranoid thinking.

After reading so many books on the subject, I was convinced he needed weekly therapy with a psychologist. I believed he needed to work through his feelings, not just discuss the effects of his medication. Every recovery model included psychosocial therapy, particularly cognitive behavioral therapy (CBT), to teach patients to respond appropriately to stimuli that made them anxious or paranoid, improving function and reducing relapse.[1] This is also referred to as psychoeducation. Because Pat still did not recognize or agree with his diagnosis, I felt that psychoeducation might be the first step in helping him to understand what schizophrenia is and bring some of his symptoms into awareness.

CBT addresses social anxiety by examining the thoughts (cognitions) that contribute to the anxiety and then gradually exposing a person to the stimulus they fear, in Pat's case social situations, in order to change the person's reaction to it. The idea is that avoidance of social situations is negative reinforcement. It reinforces the idea that there is something significantly terrifying about social situations, thus ensuring that over time Pat is less likely to enter into them. If he could expose himself to the discomfort of social situations he would gradually get used to it. Meanwhile, addressing the thoughts that make him so averse to social interaction and strangers is good practice for when those feelings rear up again.[2] CBT is essentially training in being your own therapist, giving you the skills to manage your own specific treatment. CBT has also been shown to be effective for schizophrenia, helping a patient pinpoint the anxieties that can trigger relapse and showing him how to strategize.[3] It's important that therapy be tailor-made to fit the patient's circumstances, which in schizophrenia can be vastly different from patient to patient. CBT includes coping strategies, social skills training, and relaxation techniques invaluable for any person. No wonder some of us can't count on one hand the number of people we know who see a psychologist. It was my hope that just going to weekly meetings with a psychologist would help Pat habituate to that social experience and that one day maybe he would be open to going to group therapy. There is so much that can be gained from talking to other people with schizophrenia. It's almost as if the illness wants him to stand alone, for it to be Pat against the world.

It wasn't sheer pessimism that had me convinced we had to be vigilant against a relapse or medication noncompliance. It was all the literature I read. Now I understood why Mom and Dad weren't pushing to add anything to

Pat's treatment plan. They hadn't read any of the books, and they were scared to face more change. They were still letting sleeping dogs lie.

"I think we should think about finding him some CBT," I told Mom.

"He's taking the medication. He's fine," she said, almost laughing at the suggestion.

"Has he ever said anything about what the medication is for?"

"Well, no."

"Do you think he really recognizes the diagnosis?"

"I suppose he does if he's taking the medication."

"If I asked him about the antipsychotic he takes, he would say he takes it for paranoid schizophrenia?"

"I don't know, Sarah. You'd have to ask him." She waved the idea away. I could see now where this was all headed.

I got the feeling that because I wasn't around anymore, I had no right to criticize. I didn't want the responsibility of dictating or changing Pat's treatment, but I couldn't understand how inaction was going to help him. Having my own social anxieties, I knew that the longer I went without facing my fear, the harder it was to do. If I spent the better part of a week at home and then had a dentist's appointment, actually keeping the appointment was almost insurmountable. I would need someone to accompany me and literally walk me to the door.

His psychiatrist had no plan to help Pat recover socially, regain friendships, and become comfortable just shopping at a grocery store without anxiety. With the amount of avoidance Pat was displaying, I worried that one day he wouldn't leave the house at all. My parents felt that Pat was fine. He had his life back, and with the medication they felt he would never be psychotic again. They didn't feel vigilance was necessary. They seemed to think I was trying to fix something that wasn't broken anymore. Mom and I argued about it. When I told Dad that Pat's treatment needed a change, he was dumbstruck. "What happened?" he asked.

"Nothing yet."

It was very confusing for him. Why would I want to intervene when I wasn't sure anything was wrong? "You worry too much, sweetie." I had sensed their denial from New York, but now I was sure of it. Of course it's much easier to see someone else's denial and not one's own.

The flight to New Orleans and the flight back were harrowing. The last few times I had flown, I was nervous, but now I was completely unhinged. I listened to every sound the plane made, certain that each one was a bad omen, the engine dying or a wing coming off. We're accelerating because we're falling! Any minute we would plummet from the sky in a spinning, fiery tragedy. I clung to Gavin's arm the whole flight. With every bump I gave him a look of absolute terror.

Each time I boarded a plane afterward, the anxiety was bigger. As soon as I bought a plane ticket, I would begin worrying over the flight. It didn't matter that it was two months away. People would quote me statistics and tell me that it was safer to fly than ride in a car. But the statistics didn't matter to me. My flight would be that one in millions that went down. Anything could happen, right? I mean, look at what happened to New Orleans. Look at what happened to Pat.

My anxiety was spilling over. It was getting on everything in my life. First it was the subway; now it was air travel. I needed a psychologist. I needed to work through my own cognitive behavioral dysfunction. Looking online for a therapist, I finally got the courage to search for the symptoms I displayed in the subway (see table 12.1).

I knew that what I was feeling was probably psychological, but I didn't believe I could panic without knowing it. There had to be some obvious stressor around, but there wasn't one. I was simply around a lot of people, and that led to panic attacks. I never had a panic attack on an airplane, but it was fueled by anxiety just the same.

I couldn't stand it anymore. Unable to manage on my own, I found a psychologist in Brooklyn. Dr. Little was a young woman with brilliant red curls

Table 12.1.   DSM-IV Criteria for a Panic Attack

A period of intense fear or discomfort in which four or more of the following symptoms occur abruptly and peak within ten minutes:
- Sweating
- Trembling or shaking
- Shortness of breath
- Feeling of choking
- Chest pain
- Palpitations, pounding heart, or accelerated heart rate
- Nausea
- Dizziness
- Fear of losing control
- Fear of dying
- Derealization (feelings of unreality) or depersonalization (being detached from oneself)
- Numbness or tingling (paresthesia)
- Chills or hot flushes

who always wore these billowy, paisley skirts. Her voice was soothing, and she was very attentive. I found it easy to open up to her.

She taught me that exposure was important, but I needed the tools to counteract the way being on the subway made me feel. Relaxation techniques were key. I felt more confident with them in my arsenal when I felt the dizziness coming on. I learned to control my breathing, and while I was busy doing that I had almost no time to think about my fear or what else was happening physiologically. Eventually I realized that months had gone by without any panic.

It took longer to get over my flying phobia because it's a costly thing to expose oneself to on a regular basis. Dr. Little helped me counteract the way my breathing would change when I was panicking. "Breath in slowly," she said, "and count to five. Now let it out slowly through your lips, like blowing on hot soup. And again."

I went home and compiled a playlist of videos taken on airplanes, both at takeoff and landing, and listened to them while trying to relax. My heart rate shot up—nothing I could do about that. I inhaled slowly, counted to five, and let it out slowly. With practice, I felt a little calmer each time I heard the airplane sounds.

Doing these breathing exercises made the rest of my body relax. The tension left my muscles, and my legs relaxed. My heart rate would still betray me, but eventually it would settle down too. I used the technique on my flight home for Christmas. It was a miracle. Before the flight even took off, I was almost too tired to stay awake. We hit a few bumps, and I reminded myself, "You're not here to fly the plane. Your job is to manage your anxiety." When Dad picked me up from the airport, I was glowing. He asked if I'd had a drink on the plane.

After a long period of settling in, I was finally proud to call myself a New Yorker. It's such an important town that you start to feel like you're living in the center of the universe. You want nothing more than to be let in, to be a permanent part of it. As my psychologist helped me to work through my panic attacks, I began to embrace the city and all it had to offer. I imagined that a psychologist could do the same thing for my brother, if we could only find one and get Pat to stick with it.

13

Survivor's Guilt

When I first moved away to New York, all Pat said to me was, "Goodbye, Sarah. I'll miss our conversations."

It was an awkward statement, but he was becoming an increasingly awkward kind of guy. I appreciated his honesty. Part of me wanted to stay just so he'd never have to miss anything.

I found it very difficult to have a relationship with Pat over the phone. He was never the most talkative person, but on the phone he's very tight-lipped. Perhaps he thought someone was listening. It was very unusual to not have him to talk to during Mom and Dad's separation. Who do you talk to about your parents if not your siblings?

Unable to change the present condition, I kept getting lost in the past. I would think about the old Pat, when we watched movies together and smoked marijuana. I remembered his laugh, his sly smile when he was being sarcastic. I rarely ever saw that smile anymore. At work, before his illness, when I would barge into his office with a stack of papers, he would turn to me, take my wrists, and shake them. Whatever I was holding would fall to the floor. Then he would look at me with a childish grin, and I would burst out laughing. Whatever urgent matter I was obsessing over was gone.

I had an overwhelming sense that I had failed him. He was my rock, the only thing that got me through a rough adolescence wrought with depression. And where was I for him now? I had left him behind. We had been in it together, survived the war that was growing up in our family, but when I stood at the edge of the battlefield and looked around, my confidant was gone. I know I didn't make him sick. I couldn't make him whole again, and yet I couldn't forgive myself for leaving him in New Orleans.

While I was battling my own anxiety demons, I couldn't help but imagine that he, the Pat I grew up with, would have been much better at living in the big city. Between the panic attacks and feeling dwarfed by the city, I was helpless. It didn't seem right that I was the one out in the world, going to graduate school. Growing up, Pat was clearly the one who handled change better. He was the fearless, mature one. He had been the one who wanted to see the world, go away to school, and get a graduate degree. I wasn't living my future. I was living his. The illness got the wrong kid.

I turned to my psychologist hoping she could help me work through these ominous feelings. "It's not just that I got through the family dysfunction without becoming sick. But I also had the same chance of inheriting whatever genes he inherited that contributed to his illness."

Dr. Little was an enthusiastic listener. She nodded a lot. "Have you ever heard of survivor's guilt?"

"I don't think so."

"It happens if a person survives a disastrous event that others don't. Many people who survived the Holocaust had trouble forgiving themselves. They couldn't understand why they made it and others didn't."

I couldn't see how my situation related to something on scale with the Holocaust. "But there wasn't a disaster," I said.

"A lot of people were diagnosed with PTSD after Hurricane Katrina. Survivor's guilt is part and parcel of posttraumatic stress."

"But we both survived the storm."

"What I mean is that you went through a series of traumatic events. The hurricane, your brother becoming sick, even your move to New York, could all be categorized as traumatic. Would you agree?"

I nodded, but it was unclear if she was in the process of diagnosing me with PTSD.

"You went through a lot together."

That's when our conversations usually turned to talk about my parents. It seemed that all Dr. Little wanted to talk about was my childhood. Although she said she specialized in cognitive behavioral therapy, our sessions weren't very pragmatic. The CBT approach is to identify pragmatic cognitions that lead to unwanted behaviors and then systematically implement new ways of thinking in order to change those behaviors. For example, if I often get anxious when I ride in a taxicab and I don't know why, a cognitive behavioral therapist would try to help me uncover the automatic thoughts or impulses that lead to my anxiety and help me train myself to focus on alternative thoughts when I get into a taxi.

In the beginning of treatment, Dr. Little helped me to uncover cognitions that amped up my anxiety when I rode the subway. But once my panic attacks were under control, she just wanted to jog through my life history every appointment. She didn't send me home with homework anymore. She wasn't having me challenge my current ways of thinking and feeling. We just talked for fifty minutes, and I left feeling a little robbed. I couldn't see how any of this was helpful to anyone who wasn't writing my biography. What was she looking for in my past? There was no secret, defining event that made me an anxious person or, for that matter, made Pat a schizophrenic.

I knew that my survivor's guilt was unfounded, but it didn't matter. I suppose an old ghost of depression still followed right on my heels. It could eat up my self-esteem in an instant. I bought into the idea that it should have been me, wanting to sacrifice myself so that Pat could be well. The only thing that kept me from wallowing in it indefinitely was the glimmer of hope that there are other people out there dealing with the same thing as me. There had to be another person with a brother or sister suffering from severe mental illness. They ran into the same roadblocks, had similar arguments with their family, felt helpless, and maybe even guilty. They didn't survive a catastrophe or a pandemic. They just made it through development without becoming sick, while their sibling was not so lucky.

I learned about the National Alliance on Mental Illness (NAMI) through an online search for "mental health support." That's where I found the Family-to-Family program. It's for family and friends of someone with mental illness. These were free group meetings that combined learning with sharing our experiences. It promised to introduce me to other families and caregivers, as well as new resources. Family-to-Family met once a week for twelve weeks, and once I finished it I could graduate to more specific groups, ones just for siblings and ones just dealing with schizophrenia.

The first day of group, they handed us a big binder and went over at least thirty handouts. These were emergency contact numbers and lists of patient's rights. It was comforting to have, although I still hated the idea of calling the police on Pat. Furthermore, these numbers were for New York patients, not Louisiana patients.

Then we broke the ice by introducing ourselves and talking about the circumstances that brought us to NAMI. Out of twenty members, there were two other women in the room who had a sibling with schizophrenia. One was a twenty-one-year-old woman whose nineteen-year-old brother had recently been diagnosed with paranoid schizophrenia. The other was an elderly woman. Her sister had been diagnosed with schizophrenia over forty years ago. Their mother had always been her sister's caregiver, but she had recently passed away. Now this woman was taking her sister into her home and was shocked by her behavior.

These women were two opposite ends of the spectrum: early life, just after diagnosis, when everything seems terrifying and surreal, and late life, after a full case history, when things might be a little more predictable and then you inherit the responsibility of caring for your sibling. I could look at the young woman fresh out of the trenches and be thankful I had gotten through that period of psychosis and diagnosis. In the case of the older woman, I imagined I would be more prepared to take Pat in if it came to that later in life.

We went over signs and symptoms of different mental illnesses, which was a little boring for me considering my background. But it was all worth it when we would share. A good dose of perspective can immediately give a person a more positive outlook. An elderly man said his fifty-two-year-old bipolar son had been off medication for two years and was doing very well. Sometimes group members reminded you of your worst fears. One couple in class had a fifteen-year-old son recently diagnosed with schizophrenia. He was convinced they were poisoning his food. The fear in their voices as they spoke was palpable.

"For what it's worth," the group leader said, "we've all been there too." Our group leader was in her forties. She was married to a man with schizophrenia. Her husband suffered from delusions of persecution much like Pat's. She said her husband had changed the locks on their apartment at least twenty times in the last decade. Her composure when she was talking about this was remarkable. She wasn't like the rest of us with our wide eyes and our dropping hearts. She was matter-of-fact. There was no shame in the way she spoke, and she wasn't worried about how scary it might sound. It was absolutely clear that she was in the driver's seat. No matter what she came home to, no matter what her husband went through, she could face it down. I wanted a piece of that.

Oftentimes it is crisis that makes us finally turn to NAMI. It can be hard to make the commitment to go to meetings. It's not unlike putting off a new diet or exercise until you start having high blood pressure. The twenty-one-year-old with the schizophrenic little brother stopped coming to group after a couple of weeks. She was a college student. Likely it was too hard to attend the NAMI class with a full-time schedule. Then again maybe she didn't find much comfort there. She had her whole life ahead of her. Her little brother wasn't under her care alone. She had her own life to live.

Then I finally appreciated why the elderly woman was so unprepared when her schizophrenic sister came to live with her. After forty years, how would she be prepared? She had followed her own path, taking responsibility for her own life all those years. What could prepare her for the sister she would inherit when their mother died? Mental illness evolves over time, and the people directly involved change with it. If I learned anything from NAMI, it is that. Treatment is so specific to the patient, no one could even begin to write an instruction manual for caregiving. Some patients don't need medication anymore later in life. Some caregivers have stringent routines, and the patient develops long-standing habits.

By the end of class, I left feeling much more confident. It wasn't just the resources they sent me home with. They had inadvertently taught me coping skills. It wasn't like talking to Dr. Little. She usually made wide, concerned eyes when I talked to her about Pat's troubles. At first it was comforting. I thought, "Good. She understands how serious all this is, how big the loss." Over time that was too much for me. I was tired of fear and consolation. Being scared of schizophrenia wasn't going to help anything.

Through NAMI, I came to believe that schizophrenia is not the end of anything. It's a beast of an illness, but it's no match for an informed caregiver. Until then, I felt I was too passive in Pat's treatment. But being active doesn't mean taking the helm. I can't control Pat, but I can always be there to support him. I can meet his fear with empathy. I can make myself a wealth of information about his illness, even if he doesn't seem to recognize that he has a mental illness. Patience and flexibility replaced the knot in my stomach.

Dr. Little didn't seem to know much about NAMI or the Family-to-Family program.

"It was a real eye-opener," I told her. "All these other people were going through the same thing, but we all faced it together. By the end, we laughed at some of the things we talked about. We were empowered. It doesn't seem like such a raw deal anymore. I think I'm past feeling guilty."

"That's wonderful," she nodded cheerfully.

"It's not that I suddenly think Pat's better off this way. It's just that stuff happens, and we just have to get through it. And we will. We've gotten through everything else." I thought she was going to launch into my childhood again, so I kept talking. "I suppose I felt a lot of pressure—not just to save Pat, but to make up for his losses. Sometimes I feel like I have to be perfect to make up for it. I worried that I would disappoint my parents. Now I think the only thing that would disappoint them is knowing that I felt that way."

"Are you going to more group meetings, or was that the last of them?"

"I'm not sure. But it's comforting to know that they're always there."

"I'm glad you recognize that you deserve the support just as much as your brother does. A lot of good comes from group meetings. I run a few addiction groups down in Coney Island."

"I think it's time I found some groups down in Louisiana. I think my parents could get a lot out of NAMI." I hesitated, not wanting to start micromanaging my parents. "At least they might take comfort knowing it's there if they need it."

Dr. Little didn't weigh in on that. Instead she launched into more questions about my parents and what they were like when I was growing up. It was strange the way she never really asked about Pat. She didn't seem to be the least bit curious about that part of my life. It felt like he was removed from my history, marginalized, unimportant. I would have to go elsewhere if I really wanted to talk about Pat and celebrate my memory of him.

14

The First Noncompliance

Pat was never secretive growing up. He always shared, as if he needed reassurance from others. Although he had withdrawn a great deal since the onset of his schizophrenia, there must have been some last vestiges of that in him. It was Mom's birthday in 2008. Pat was supposed to go to dinner with her. He showed up agitated, jittery, and wild-eyed. He told her his feelings about being spied on by some unknown agent. "I've stopped taking my medication," he said. "I can see things more clearly now. I *am* being watched."

They didn't go out to dinner that night. Mom stayed the night at Pat's house. When Mom called to tell me what had happened, I slumped down on the floor. There wasn't much to say. When I hung up, I burst into tears. I knew this could happen, but it didn't matter. It had almost been a year since I moved to Brooklyn. Pat was off his meds and floridly psychotic, and I was huddled on the floor of my apartment like a blubbering mass.

There had long been a hole in the wooden fence that surrounded his backyard. I'm not sure if it was damage from Katrina or just the natural decay of the old, untreated wood. Pat was now certain that someone was filming him through the hole. When he'd walk up to it, nothing was there, but that's because the person would run away. He thought it had to be the neighbors doing it. If not them, they had given someone access to their yard in order to videotape him.

Mom stayed with him for several days, twenty-four hours a day. She could barely sleep because Pat didn't. She would doze off and wake up to find him in the foyer putting on his shoes. "I just want to talk to them, Mom."

Her biggest fear was that he would confront the neighbors. It was a young family, renting the shotgun house next door. They had a little girl, kindergarten age. It was reasonable to think that if they felt threatened and called the police, Pat would be forcibly hospitalized. We weren't against hospitalization, but he'd have to be found harmful in order to be committed. We didn't believe he was dangerous, just delusional and manic.

Mom stayed with him almost a week without any respite. There was no convincing him to take his medication again. All he wanted to talk about was the idea that he was being watched and who he could talk to for answers. Finally she was able to convince him to come stay at her house out in the country. We grew up in that house. It was not only familiar, but fairly secluded. Pat still didn't sleep there, but he no longer talked about being videotaped. All the neighboring homes were hundreds of feet away from Mom's house. She had a wire fence that no one could hide behind. When he smoked cigarettes, he would look around the yard warily, but there were no other people around. All you can find in that yard is turtles, snakes, squirrels, and some large water birds that scope out the pond for fresh fish. Once in a blue moon you'll see a rabbit or a deer.

Dad brought most of Pat's clothing to him. It seemed he was moving in with Mom. After two months, he still refused to see his psychiatrist or take his medication. There seemed to be no end in sight.

Mom kept several dogs, all of which Pat had named. We saw them a lot in high school, but much less when we went to college. I always suspected Pat missed them when he moved away, although he said nothing of it. He lived with an old dog in New Orleans, but she died just weeks before we found out about his medication noncompliance. It was a complicated death. She slowly lost the use of her back legs, then her ability to hold her bowels, and then her will to eat. It was a long, insidious way to go.

Taking the country dogs outside and feeding them was not only a simple responsibility; it gave Pat a reason to get up every day. The routine was something he latched onto, and it brought a sense of stability to his life.

As it started getting warmer outside, his energy level dropped. He would sleep in and not take the dogs out for their morning run. His anxiety decreased as well. It was as if he was too tired to worry anymore. He would sleep all day and get up in the evening.

Mom tried having many discussions with him to get him to see a psychiatrist, but it wasn't until she threatened to make him move out on his own that he ceded. "I'll go see a doctor, but I want to see a new one. I'm not going back to Hollis."

"I understand," Mom told him. "I don't want you to see someone you don't trust."

That's when it became clear how important it is for a schizophrenic to trust his therapist. The stakes are so high for the patient, whether real or imagined. If a cancer patient thought his doctor was a quack, he'd certainly get a second opinion. It should be no different for a mentally ill patient.

I'd had my doubts before about my own therapist. My psychologist, Dr. Little, had trouble addressing my specific needs as a sibling of a person with schizophrenia, but it wasn't of dire consequence. I just supplemented our sessions with my NAMI group. Doubt in therapy for a schizophrenic has repercussions that tie into the patient's very own paranoid delusions. At first Pat seemed to like that Dr. Hollis was close to him in age, but perhaps it was inexperience itself that caused the rift between them. Whatever the cause, Pat was given several referrals.

His new psychiatrist lived nearly an hour away in New Orleans. The biggest selling point for Dr. Russell was that he was the father of identical twins, one of whom had schizophrenia while the other did not. I was relieved to hear this, imagining some large-scale treatment plan that would one day bring Pat back into the light.

Dr. Russell met with Mom and Pat separately and then called them in together. "I'm going to start him out on the same medication he used to take, since you said he responded well before he stopped taking it. The difference is that this is an extended release version. You should feel a lot less groggy while taking this kind. Come back in a few weeks and tell me how they're working for you. If you have any allergic reactions, call me right away."

"Allergic reactions?" Mom asked.

"Hives, swelling of the tongue, difficulty breathing."

Pat didn't say whether he agreed to take the pills or not, but he didn't make a verbal protest either.

In the car, Mom held her breath. "So," she sighed, "what did you think?"

"I think it's fine."

She waited a moment. "You like him? You'll see him once a month?"

He sighed begrudgingly. "Once a month?"

She nodded.

"Yeah, I guess that's okay."

Six months passed. He took a room in Mom's house, my childhood bedroom actually. He had no intention of returning to the suburbs of New Orleans or to work. He spent most of his days with the dogs. Sometimes he watched TV or cleaned the swimming pool.

He was very tight-lipped when I saw him. When he spoke, it was almost too quiet for me to make out what he was saying. It annoyed him if I asked him to repeat himself. It seemed to cheer him up having Gavin there. He didn't spend any time with men his own age anymore.

I'd never seen so much hair on his face in his life. He was growing a beard. He always complained he couldn't grow one. I guess the trick was letting half a year go by. Mom said he grew it because he hated being in the bathroom. She had to bargain with him to get him to shower and shave every day. It took me by surprise. This from the guy who always used to tell me that if I just washed my hands thirty seconds longer, I might save hundreds of people from the flu every year.

"He looks clean enough," Gavin said.

"He's not. His hair is dirty," Mom told him.

"If the medication works, shouldn't he be managing his hygiene?" I asked.

"We see Dr. Russell in a couple of weeks. I plan on talking to him about it," she said.

On the medication he was less anxious, but he still had suspicions about being watched. Dr. Russell said that if the medication was working properly he would not feel that way. He felt that six months was plenty of time to wait for the medication to be effective. It was time to try something new. Pat began taking another second-generation antipsychotic, the same one he had taken in the past when Dr. Hollis thought he might be bipolar. I was surprised to learn that many of the same drugs used to treat schizophrenia are also prescribed for bipolar. While it's unclear exactly how it works, adjusting dopamine in the brain seems to have an array of benefits in treating severe mental illness.

While I liked Dr. Russell's proactive approach to finding the right medication, switching to another drug was frightening to me. When Mom said they would have to start with a low dose and increase it slowly up to a full dose, I worried he'd grow more paranoid in the meantime. Little did I know that would be the best time of the year for him.

He started working again for Dad's real estate agency, this time remotely from home. A spare bedroom was turned into a home office with a desk and file cabinets. Calls were forwarded from the office to his phone line, and a computer was set up so he could access the office's network. Despite the fact that he was not leaving the house, the fact that he was working again bolstered the idea that he was in recovery.

Then as the colder months crept in things began to change. Pat was sleep-eating again. Mom was the first to actually witness Pat walk into the kitchen, make some food, leave it out, and return to bed. She didn't realize he was asleep at first and would try to engage with him. Talking to a sleepwalker must be a strange experience for most people, but on the spectrum of Pat's strange behavior, this was about as frightening as a kitten. "He wasn't making a lot of sense," Mom said. "I got him to turn around and go back to his room. A few minutes later he was sleeping again."

If waking up in the morning and finding food spoiling on the counter is frustrating, when Pat denies that he's the culprit it's even more annoying. Mom cleaned up the mess. He wouldn't be getting up until the afternoon.

Dr. Russell said the sleepwalking was normal. While not everyone with schizophrenia sleepwalks, it had long been a part of Pat's disease. Dr. Russell wanted to give him something to help him sleep, but he wanted to wait until Pat was on a full dose of the antipsychotic. However reasonable, this still annoyed me. Still feeling like we were holding a lit stick of dynamite, I had no patience for these slow and mysterious antipsychotics.

By Christmastime, Pat was on a full dose of antipsychotic, but there was an upswing in his delusional thinking. He was more energetic and talkative. He didn't sleep much. Soon he was having delusions about Mom's next-door neighbors. He came to Mom with his concerns: "I keep finding things moved or broken."

"Pat, you sleepwalk. You move things all the time. I can't tell you how many times I get up in the morning and you've left bowls and food and milk out on the counter. One night I got up and the fridge was open."

He studied her face quietly and then said, "I still think we should call the police."

"We're not calling the police, Pat."

"Why not?"

"Because nobody is coming into the house. If you call the police, they will come and take you."

He didn't want to speak to her about it after that, and he retreated to his bedroom. The discussion never became heated, but it left Mom feeling uneasy.

When I came to visit for the holidays, Mom had to turn off the alarm system to let me into the house. "But you're home. Why is it on?" I asked.

"He likes it that way," she shrugged.

Next to the front door was a cardboard box. Covering its top was a red and green tablecloth. Walking into the kitchen, I saw several more boxes piled in front of the back door. It was also adorned with a holiday tablecloth. "What's that?"

"It's a box of shelves." A long box, it sat about a foot off the floor and snug against the length of the door.

"How do you get outside?"

"He prefers to go out of the garage instead of using the backdoor."

"Mom, what's going on here?"

"He thinks people are coming into the house when he's sleeping."

"Coming into the house for what?"

"He doesn't know," she shrugged.

Pat walked through, going outside to smoke. I hadn't seen him in months, and all he did was nod at me as he went out. His hair and beard were longer and greasy. His clothes were worn and baggy.

"Mom?" I shook my head.

"I told him that things are going to change, but I'm waiting until after Christmas."

"Why?"

"So we can have a relaxing Christmas."

"How is this relaxing?"

"Come on, Sarah, I'm the one who has to live here with him."

"Do you have to turn off the alarm every time you go in and out?"

She nodded. "I set it off a few times. It's awfully loud. That's why I told him I'm sick of it. We're not doing this in the new year."

"When did this start?"

"Around November." She poured glasses of wine for us both.

"You decorated the boxes for Christmas?" Mom gave me a look that was both leery and cheerful. I thought, "She's going to go crazy too if this keeps up."

Other than to see his psychiatrist once a month, Pat never left the house. Mom and Dad ran errands for him. He'd make a list; Mom complained of the cost. He didn't give her money to cover the expense unless she explicitly asked him to. All her utility bills doubled, and he didn't help with those either.

For Mom, running his errands was the alternative to arguing with him to do it himself. Obstinate, he would complain that she was going to the store anyway. I told her that she should make him come with her, but she said he wasn't interested in doing that either.

Dad saw getting groceries for Pat as a failsafe. "I don't want him driving around while he's on that medication. He gets so groggy."

"The medication warns about drinking while taking it, not about operating machinery like a car. Plenty of people on antipsychotics go about their usual day without being *assisted* with everything."

"Well, look at him. He looks homeless. What if someone calls the police?"

"It's not a crime to look homeless." I thought about it a moment. "Maybe he'd be more likely to clean up if he ever left the house." I was caught between a rock and a hard place. I wanted Pat to leave the house. Letting him stay in all the time negatively reinforced his fears of the outside world. What would he do if he didn't have anyone around to cater to his needs?

"Hopefully it won't always be that way," Mom told me.

I didn't expect Pat to make any changes on his own. I had already been shocked at how unabashedly and wholeheartedly he depended on our parents. I watched him ask Mom to get him some more cigarettes. When she said it would have to wait until the following day, he stalked off insolently like a child.

Pat didn't eat all day. He'd begin drinking wine around five or six o'clock at night. He'd become more talkative, sometimes standing in the kitchen with me for a while before returning to his room or going out to smoke. He was nearly stumbling about by the time he ate his evening meal, which consisted of a frozen dinner. "Pasta," Mom said, "that's all he wants to eat."

"Is he supposed to be drinking?"

"The alcohol just makes him drowsy. He's usually very careful about how much he has. Too much will make him sleepwalk, and he hates that. It's the medication, Sarah. We keep changing the dosage, and then he doesn't know his limit."

"I don't think he should be drinking at all."

"Well you tell him that then."

"Just stop buying it for him," I fumed. I wanted someone to take the reins of Pat's treatment, while my parents weren't interested in making waves. It felt like we were working at odds. It's impossible to say which technique is best until you view the decisions from hindsight. Of course it's important to look to the future, like I did, but that can be counterintuitive when strange delusions arise and evolve each week. Dealing with each day as it comes, the way our parents did, had its benefits. "It's schizophrenia," Mom told me. "It's unpredictable. You can't follow a plan."

"Yes you can. I met families in NAMI who had action plans." I said it, but I couldn't even imagine where we would begin. With the delusions, Pat still wasn't even stable.

Mom sighed and rolled her eyes. We weren't on the same page. We were coming apart at the seams. The year 2008 came and went with moderate improvement, and then a descent into medicated madness. This must have been what Dr. Hollis meant when he told me that Pat's symptoms could flare up. We were supposed to be his support when that happened, but was Mom supporting him? Was it right to accommodate his fears? Was it right for all his needs to be taken care of for him so that he never had to leave the house? I had no choice but to acquiesce with my parents. After all, I was the one who would be returning to Brooklyn, the absent caregiver, and he was living with my mom. And what did I know about what was best for Pat? Someone who sees him every day is likely much more qualified to assess his treatment. I was at a loss.

Dad got Pat a beautiful new guitar for Christmas, but he wasn't interested in it. He wasn't even excited about it. We had to ask him several times on Christmas Day to come open it. Pat didn't play the guitar anymore. He wasn't using the phone or Internet either—he was cut off from the world. He didn't buy cards or presents for anyone for any reason. He wore the same clothes every day. It took a great deal of bargaining on Mom's part to get him to wash the clothes while he was taking a shower once a month. Then the showers stopped altogether.

Mom had just convinced Pat to stop piling boxes in front of the doors when he began voicing a new concern. "First he was showering in the dark," Mom told me. "He wouldn't turn on any lights. Now he says he thinks there's a camera or something in the showerhead. He doesn't want to go in there at all. I've offered to have it changed, but he says no."

Mom had a plumber at her house helping her to remodel the master bathroom. Pat seemed suspicious about having a stranger in the house. Workers had been to the house before, but this was different. The plumber was around nearly every day for a month.

Working at home became too much for Pat. A client had an urgent problem and left him a series of messages. Because Pat didn't get up until the afternoon, he didn't take care of it until after office hours. He seemed relieved to stop working.

Dad replaced the showerhead in his bathroom, but Pat still refused to use it. "It doesn't make a difference," he claimed without any further explanation.

Dr. Russell was worried about the rash of breakthrough symptoms. Mom said they were moving on to a relatively new antipsychotic, which many of Dr. Russell's patients had very good results taking. "He's got to step down from the antipsychotic gradually. He'll keep taking the antidepressant though."

"He's depressed?" I asked, not knowing he was taking the drug.

"I talked to him. He said he's not sad but anxious. It was Dr. Russell's suggestion to add an antidepressant. He said a lot of patients get down, especially after they've tried so many drugs without improvement."

My heart sank. I hadn't considered this before. He seemed so blank the last time I saw him. Was I too blind to see he was sad? "Does he seem sad to you, Mom?"

"No, honey. Look, we have an agreement. If he feels down, especially if he feels like hurting himself, he will come talk to me about it."

I was relieved. Pat and Mom always had a close relationship. That bond was a lifeline. What did Dr. Russell see in him that made him prescribe an antidepressant? Maybe he was as tired as the rest of us. The different medications, not having a job anymore—maybe he even noticed the strain it put on Mom and Dad. It was a bittersweet revelation. Although the medication wasn't perfect, Pat had a glimmer of insight. Instead of having insight into how far he'd come, how integral his communicativeness and open-mindedness were to getting him help, he recognized himself as a burden and saw the time and effort the family was putting forth to help him.

15

Letters Never Sent

I always thought that even though I moved away, Pat would always be available to talk on the phone. But he didn't use the phone anymore, and soon I was beginning to feel like an only child. If I called him, he would neither answer nor return the call. He didn't answer text messages. He deleted all his old e-mail addresses. To him the Internet was too much exposure. It felt like a conduit for people to spy on him. Thus long-distance communication was on his terms. When I was in a room with him, I would talk feverishly, needing to get it all out before I returned to Brooklyn. I'm sure it was overwhelming for him, but he never let on. My once confidant, and here I was now smothering him with my attention.

I used to share everything with him. Every time something happened to me, big or small, my first reaction was to tell Pat. Knowing that he was taking an antidepressant, I wanted to talk to him about that too and compare our feelings. While I was never diagnosed with depression and never took antidepressants, sadness was something I knew all too well. Maybe I would have some words of wisdom for him. Then again, I was feeling so isolated that I was having my own trouble staying ahead of my lurking depression. I worried that if I brought it up, he wouldn't know what I was talking about. Maybe he wouldn't be happy knowing that I had so much information about his therapy. In 2009, almost two years since his first medication noncompliance and moving in with Mom, I realized that the flow of communication between Pat and me had shut down. Having not found a medication that he was particularly responsive to, Dr. Russell didn't feel that the schizophrenia was stabilized. So it didn't seem like the right time to call Pat up and say, "I want us to talk more. I miss our long conversations. I feel I have so much to tell you since I moved to New York, and there's never a great time to say it."

I dreamed of Pat on a regular basis. Not like the nightmares I used to have during the onset of his illness—he wasn't in danger in these dreams. These may have been worse. I had dreams that he was perfectly healthy. He was the old Pat, smiling and sarcastic. Maybe we were at some family function and he was hanging out with me, telling me jokes, making fun of something Dad said. Then I would wake up, slowly letting the morning wash over me. I felt happy, and he felt near to me. Then I remembered it was only a dream. He was back in New Orleans, struggling to recover from schizophrenia, not leaving the house and full of suspicion.

I threw my worries onto Dr. Little. I told her about my dreams, dreams I never wanted to be torn away from. Those are the real nightmares, the kind that latch onto your longings, not just your fears. I told her that I felt adrift at sea without him. I didn't know how to reopen the flow of communication. "Do you think he knows? Do you think he remembers how close we were? Do you think he misses me?"

Dr. Little was a deer in the headlights. "Ah . . ." she trailed off. I often felt I had to force my psychologist to discuss my brother with me. "So how is he doing on his medication now?"

"There's really not any progress."

"That must be very hard on you."

"It's been particularly hard on our parents." I explained all the work they did caring for him.

When I was done, she looked at her watch and said, "I think we have to stop for today."

That was the rift that eventually led to the end of my therapy. Weeks later, I told her I was ready "to take off the training wheels," and Dr. Little gave me her blessing. It seemed wrong that she was happy for me to leave therapy. I guess I had always been waiting for her to turn to me and tell me that I was finished—she'd just say, "Sarah, you're ready. You don't need me anymore." But I appreciated that she didn't try to get me to stay either. Her faith in me gave me more confidence.

I knew that much of cognitive behavioral therapy meant doing a great deal of work at home. I was managing my anxiety. The most valuable thing I learned from Dr. Little was that everything is a work in progress. If I found myself sweating the small stuff, I would go back to practicing my breathing and reminding myself to let things go. Having fear on a plane or anxiety in a public space wasn't necessarily a setback. It was an opportunity to break out the relaxation tools I'd learned and practice a little emotional self-management. I even started enjoying myself in new social situations.

While I was climbing around in my own brain trying to make it the comfortable and idyllic place I always wanted it to be, I found a hole, a place I would go to feel bad. It was a place that used to be filled by my best friend and roommate.

Everyone warned me that Pat would never be the same after his onset. Each time he descended into active-phase psychosis, it would put distance between who he was and who he had been. I didn't believe them at first, but it was true. Doctors made no promises: "Don't expect him to wake up tomorrow and be the old Pat."

But he was still there, even if he was very different. There is no guidebook for grieving someone alive. It felt unfair to call myself bereaved. Anyone who has lost a loved one would resent that. I still had a brother. I needed to find a way to cope with my grief and the guilt that accompanied it. It was a journey that would take me deep into the heart of my own depression.

I decided to deal with my immediate sadness by writing letters to Pat. There were so many things I couldn't say to him, and he was never one for "mushy" talk. This was my opportunity to pour my heart out. I never meant to send them. I knew it was a method for finding closure in situations where closure was more or less impossible, but I was surprised at the relief it gave me.

February 9, 2008
Dear Pat,

You still aren't doing well, although you've been on this new medication for two weeks. Writing this letter is almost a replacement for a real interaction, because you're so unwell at the moment that everything I say to you is misconstrued. You're piecing together non sequiturs to feed your delusions. I can't tell you anything that you would truly understand.

Winter in New York City isn't as cold this year. The week I moved here, there was a high of about fourteen degrees. See, if I told you that over the phone right now you'd think it was code or a clever way of avoiding the issue that only you believe is at hand. You believe your neighbors are stalking you, neighbors neither you nor I have ever met before. I've been reading like crazy to find out more information, any news that might help us care for you. There are never answers, just pointers, sneaky ways of going around your illness, none of them certain to work.

I saw A Beautiful Mind *last night. Remember when we saw it together in the theater at the matinee on Riverview? When you were twenty or twenty-one. I was eighteen years old. I remember crying so much. I remember feeling so much when I watched that film. It's pathetic now. Or ironic. We sat in that theater, and there was no way to know that one of us would be afflicted one day, that one day you wouldn't know what was real anymore. And how do we get your feet back on the ground? Everything is always so simple in movies. They leap forward in time and everything is changed, better, fine.*

Your doctor says that when schizophrenics get older their symptoms diminish. He said you may not need meds at all. It's something to do with chemical changes or hormone changes in the brain. I think it's just a miracle. But not helpful. Not to us right now. We'd be in our seventies then. My greatest fear is growing old and you turning to me one day and saying, "I've missed it all. My life has passed me by." I don't know how to help you get what you want out of life. I don't know if you want anything. I don't know if you're satisfied. There could be years of research telling me that you're perfectly happy, that you don't want anything else from life, and I would still have this doubt in my heart. Take your medicine.

Love always,
Sarah

I put the letter in a large, unsealed envelope and put it on my bookcase. I marveled for a moment at the idea that one day Pat would be perfectly well, with insight into his schizophrenia. I'd give him this envelope, with however many letters I had written over the years. He would laugh and cry. I had to put that idea out of my head.

I looked at the envelope on the shelf. It wasn't real communication if I never sent the letter, but it didn't matter. I felt better. "That's enough," I told myself. I finally got to tell him how helpless I felt in the face of his mental illness, although he doesn't recognize that he has one. Soon I found myself writing to him just to reminisce.

August 8, 2008

There's stuff I want to say that I never quite get the chance to tell you. Thank you for visiting with Gavin and me last weekend while we were in town—for breaking your routine to sit on the porch with us and talk. I miss our talks.

Remember when we were kids and Billy Callard told us that we'd get the flu if we made our bodies hot and cold at the same time? It was wintertime and we didn't want to go back to school after Christmas break. So we got a bucket of hot water, put it by the swimming pool, and dunked our arms down into each of them at once. I remember looking at each other and debating how long we were supposed to do it. Later that day we weren't feeling sick, so I took a cold shower. It was miserable. We didn't get sick, but I think we still faked it the next morning.

Surely there was some overarching reason we didn't want to go back to school. I don't remember discussing it specifically. We just threw ourselves into the task of getting sick. Were we avoiding the schoolwork? Were we avoiding teachers or other kids? I was so self-conscious, I'm sure I feared my classmates the most. I remember getting heartburn for days before we'd go back to class. The end of summer was the hardest. Three months to myself and then back to the lion's den. Young girls can be so catty. It's taken me my whole life to realize that people aren't busy observing and criticizing me. They're going on with their own lives, not worried about me. In seventh grade, though, people really were watching, judging, and being ugly, because they were so insecure themselves.

I'm trying to get over that still. Even in graduate school, it's so hard for me to talk to new people. I kind of resent my classmates when I watch them hit it off so quickly. I did make one friend in class, but he turned out to be nuts. He started following me around everywhere and asking me inappropriate questions. (Where's my older brother when I need him?)

I downloaded a new album on my computer. I was looking for something to help me study. I got Bach's Brandenburg concertos performed by the Orchestra of the Age of Enlightenment. I remember how much you liked Bach. The music makes me feel close to you. That's why I stopped writing my essay and wrote this letter to you instead.

Love,
Sarah

Having parents go through a divorce once you're an adult is a tricky event. I went through all the same resentfulness and misgivings that a younger person would have, but they faded away very quickly. I just wanted our parents to be happy, and I knew that they hadn't been for a long time. I looked forward to time passing and their wounds healing. What I hadn't considered was that they would be interested in dating. The separation was so sudden and the divorce very amicable. The idea that they would move on and be ready for a new romantic relationship shocked me. Somehow it made me feel second rate. Our parents would move on and forget about their old family. They'd think of us as just some mistake they made when they were young.

I talked to other people about it, but most had parents who had divorced when they were children. Their lives were much different than mine. I even felt guilty that I was so torn up about it. Imagine how they felt when they were only children going through it. In my heart I knew the only person I could talk to about it was Pat. He could relate and give me advice. But that was the old Pat. When I tried talking to him about it now, he seemed disinterested. It was as if his mind was set on more important things, probably still worrying over his delusions. I decided to write it down instead.

January 12, 2009
Dear Pat,

Look, there's something I've been meaning to talk to you about because you're the only person who would understand. Now that the divorce is final, Dad's living the life of a bachelor. He's interested in an old colleague. Mom's interested in an old high school flame. Neither seems very happy that the other is moving on, and yet they're moving on themselves. It's not that I don't want them to be happy. I just don't want them to rush into something new. I imagine them remarrying. Spending holidays with their new, maybe even younger families—it just makes me feel like I was part of the practice family. My family was a mistake, but they'll love their new family better. Their lives will be happier, simpler, better. I feel defective, replaced. I know you don't feel that way, or at least you said as much. Maybe you've already faced those feelings when they separated, or maybe you just don't worry about this sort of thing anymore.

I feel like a teenager writing you a letter, complaining about how unfair life is. We know it's unfair. Who knows that better than you? I know what you would say. You'd say, "Sarah, don't make it all about you." I guess a lot of my identity is wrapped up in my family, even if I never thought of it that way before. It's really important to me that I feel like I'm a part of something that counts. I'm happy we've gotten to where we are, no matter how things turned out. I gave it my all, as a daughter and a sister, and I'd do it again.

Maybe I just have trouble accepting change. I can't control what Mom or Dad do. I can only control how I react. I'll try to be as flexible for them as I have been with you all this time.

Love always,
Sarah

Through writing these letters, I found myself sorting through a lot of my feelings. In trying to explain the way I felt, I could discover the real root of my emotions. I used to turn to Pat for advice, and here I was beginning to give it to myself. He had been such a positive influence in my life that he laid the groundwork. There was now a rational voice in my head helping me cope and be honest with myself.

Then I received a call from an old friend that sent me into a tailspin.

"Sarah, I don't know if you heard, but I thought it was important to tell you exactly how it happened."

"What's happened?"

"I know you were pretty close with Coach Cam." Cameron Holt was my very insightful swim coach up until high school. "He's passed away."

"What are you talking about?" Coach was only about fifty years old.

"He hung himself in his backyard."

I tried to speak but choked.

"His wife and son found him."

I remembered his son. He was just a baby when I left for high school. "Wait, I don't understand."

"I don't think anyone really understands."

"He was sad?" I never knew. I could never tell.

"I guess so."

"Thank you for calling me."

I sat stunned in my living room. I knew I should call someone, but I couldn't move. How did I not know that something was wrong? I had been depressed and suicidal while I was on the swim team. When I was thirteen, it was perhaps the worst year for me. Was he sad then, too? I knew he saw that I was the type of girl who was often too hard on herself, but was it that he saw some of himself in me?

I had thought of him several times in passing since I had moved to the city. One often wonders what old acquaintances would think if they knew you were living in New York City. That was all. I never imagined he was anything but content. He had a family of five, and he was still teaching at my old school. He was probably teaching the same course, coaching the same teams, and telling the same jokes. Then he wasn't. He was dead. The school and his family asked that the circumstances of his death not be publicized, but somehow that felt dishonest. He was suicidal. We didn't know. That was important. How could I honor his memory if I didn't realize the depression that ruled his life?

I called Mom and asked her to put Pat on the phone. He came begrudgingly. "Coach hung himself," I told Pat over the phone.

"Hmm," was all he said.

"I can't believe it." There was a long pause. He didn't seem very interested in the news.

"Well, we haven't seen him in years."

"He just didn't seem like the type of person who would commit suicide."

"I don't know. I don't know him that well."

Coach Cam had been his coach too. Why didn't he feel like he knew him? We left the conversation at that. I felt a little ridiculous for calling him in the first place. It was a surprise that he wasn't really engaged in the conversation. There was no impact for him. Perhaps he felt like it was just gossip. He must not have thought of the man much over the years. It's something I've noticed since the onset of his illness. There is a lack of personal history. He doesn't reminisce or feel any ownership of things that he's done or that might have happened to him. He doesn't use past events in his life in order to relate to new events. Some things from childhood he doesn't remember at all. Episodic or biographical memory can be impaired in schizophrenia and is considered a negative symptom. It ties into an overall lack of self-awareness that includes not recognizing that he has a mental illness and not realizing that he hasn't practiced hygiene in months.

After we spoke, I felt as though I still had more to say. I couldn't put my finger on it, but I felt there was a very important lesson to be learned here. I started writing Pat a letter I'd never send, but then I crumpled it up. I didn't have more to say to him. He couldn't be my guide when it came to suicide and depression. I needed to write to myself, search my own heart to find the lesson. For some reason the letter started off in a hypercritical way, and I knew almost immediately that something was amiss:

Dear me,

You've come a long way since middle school, when sadness was all you could wrap your head around. It was indulgent, in a way, to think of life as hard and unfriendly, then placating yourself by believing you could just give it all up.

I stopped writing and read what I wrote. It almost sounded like I was accusing myself of being spoiled or selfish—not a very tolerant way to start a conversation about such a serious subject. I remember what I learned in psychology class about handling my emotions with respect and in a nonjudgmental way. I started again:

Dear me,

I know you've fought long and hard to stay one step ahead of your depression. It presses itself into your back sometimes, and you just fall into it. While it will always be lurking in your shadow . . .

Wait, that didn't sound right. For some reason I had always assumed that sadness would always be a part of my life. In a way, I liked it about myself. It made me careful, conscientious, and sensitive to others. Maybe depression wasn't hanging on to me, but rather I was hanging on to it. But why? Would I suddenly be a bad person if I wasn't morose? I could think of plenty of people who were sensitive, friendly beings without lapses into depression. That's when it hit me. Being sad never truly served me in any way. It made me feel isolated and alone. Why was I doing this to myself? I wrote, *Sometimes you sink into sadness because you deserve it. You've made a mistake or failed someone close to you. Sometimes you just can't stand to be around yourself.*

Do I hate myself? That can't be true. I'm constantly looking for ways to improve myself, tackling my anxiety and trying to be open to new experiences. I like me. I think I'm worth a lot. If that's true, then who is this judgmental person in my head who's always beating me up? Why am I so hard on myself, like the whipping girl of some fascist dictator?

I started to see a pattern in my life. I didn't just become depressed suddenly. Instead it was a cycle that I fed myself into. I would have a setback of some kind. Instead of accepting that setback for what it was, I would heap it onto a pile of perceived shortcomings. I would count it as one more thing that meant I was no good, just garbage. And the rest of the world, everyone that I loved, would be better off without me. I even beat myself up for being a coward when I felt I couldn't face suicide. The cycle would never end if I didn't stop participating. I was helping negative feelings swallow me whole.

I crumpled up the page and started a new letter.

Dear me,

It's not you. You don't feel like you're flawed, helpless, worthless, or a waste. That voice in your head is just some amalgam of every jerk, every bully, every person who didn't judge you fairly. You don't have to let them guide your life anymore. It doesn't matter what they think. You know you are worth quite a lot. They can't control you. You are free.

It would take time, surely. I would have to keep reminding myself that I like me. I would need to think of some new personal affirmations I could bring to mind before the depression ball started rolling. But it was liberating to finally realize that I didn't hate myself. I felt sure I could be my own safety net now. I trusted myself.

I understood what my dad meant when he said I had nothing to be depressed about. Sure, he didn't handle his suicidal thirteen-year-old very well, but I can understand how the revelation of my depression blindsided him. I think the world takes for granted that people are aware of themselves. A good person may not know they're good. How many people truly know how charming, funny, smart, or caring they really are? Self-image can be light-years away from the real perception people have of that person. What's more is that I am surrounded by people who love me and even tell me on a regular basis that I mean a great deal to them. I knew it would take vigilant work to rebuild my self-image to be more accurate, but I would do the work. I owed it to myself and the people who loved me. Whether I wrote more letters, kept a journal, or blogged, writing was helping me to untangle a whole wealth of mysteries in my life. I felt closer to my family, to Pat, and even to myself.

We'll never know what was going through Coach's head at the time of his death. He was an amazing teacher who made a great impression on my life. He's a good voice to hear in the back of my head when I feel like I want to withdraw from a challenge. I appreciate his attempt to break through the front I put up and help me come out of my shell. I know he would be proud of me for not giving up, for getting off the bench and facing my fear. That is how I honor him.

16

No Family Is an Island

Five years after the diagnosis, Pat and his psychiatrist Dr. Russell were still on an epic search to find the right drug cocktail. By 2011, several had given him allergic reactions. One made his mouth and lips swell. Another made him break out in a rash on his arms, although Mom maintained that it was probably poison ivy he got while cleaning up the yard. If Pat decided a drug wasn't working for him, he would vehemently refuse to take it or to revisit it again later. At least he was willing to give them a try in the first place.

Mom was noticeably worn down from taking care of Pat. I could tell she was down. It was very hard for her to convince him to pitch in around the house or pay for his groceries. There was so little progress and so much dependence over the years, and it seemed like there was no end in sight. Reading books and talking with Dr. Russell wasn't enough. She needed support.

Mom found a Family-to-Family meeting at her local NAMI affiliate. Although he could have found his own affiliate closer to home, Dad went with her to the meetings. After most meetings, Mom would call me and talk about what she had learned. She got feedback from other families that set her mind at ease.

When I spoke to Dad about the meetings, he kept saying how lucky he felt. "So many of their loved ones have had violent outbursts. We're lucky. Things could be so much worse." I try to keep that little dose of perspective in mind when the outlook seems bleak.

After the twelve-week course ended, their positivity started to fade away. They were back to playing the waiting game, starting Pat on a new medication. Dad threw himself headlong into work, but Mom didn't have a job. Living with Pat day in and day out compounded her frustration. "He never wants to do anything. He feels like I nag him constantly. I'm beginning to think I did something wrong. Maybe I should have asked more of him growing up."

"You didn't have to, Mom. He used to pick up after himself. He used to pitch in."

"Now he doesn't do anything." I understood her frustration. The person Pat used to be still seemed largely lost.

When your family member has a severe mental illness, you often find yourself impatient with their treatment. Pat's schizophrenia was not very responsive to most antipsychotics, and his social phobia didn't help anything either. When I visited I saw that he had put up a lot of sheets on the walls of his room. He used one to cover the window, although he already had blinds. He had taken another and wrapped it around his ceiling fan. It was held in place by a bungee cord. "He thinks there are cameras. He hardly lets me into his room." Mom shook her head. Obviously he was having breakthrough positive symptoms.

Waiting for his doctor to find a medication to bring him to baseline sanity was excruciating. Schizophrenia is like a big lock with millions of tiny tumblers. Getting them all into place can't be rushed. But if Mom couldn't do anything about that, she could do something about the other families out there like her own.

"So I found myself a psychologist and I started seeing her about a week ago."

"I think that's a great idea." I had worried that Mom was becoming depressed, and even if she wasn't, I thought having someone to talk to would help her.

"I also signed up to teach the next Family-to-Family course at NAMI. I'll be assisting a woman who's done it the last few years, and hopefully soon I'll be able to take over for her," she told me.

"You're kidding," I said. I was excited that she was so committed to helping others. She made so many connections when she took the NAMI course herself, I thought it would be a good social outlet for her. She had never taught before, and I admired the self-confidence it took for her to take such a big step.

"Really, I am. I'm even a little nervous about it."

"Don't be nervous, Mom. They're just like you. Everybody there is just like us."

"It's funny, when I was in the course myself, I kept finding myself talking about you a lot."

"About me?"

"About how you studied psychology so you can help us with Pat. So many people don't have siblings who take part in their treatment. Some don't know anything about schizophrenia or bipolar or whatever their brother or sister has."

"That's sweet, Mom, but you don't have to brag to them about me," I chuckled.

"I know. You're right, sweetie. This time I'm going to talk more about Pat. Every person with schizophrenia is different. I want to tell them about this one."

She was right. We spent so many years keeping Pat's illness to ourselves. With the exception of Uncle Larry, we didn't even tell the rest of the family right away. I told myself that we didn't see the extended family very much anyway. They never called or visited Pat. I'm not sure if they knew that he had finished college the year before the diagnosis. Eventually they did start asking after him. I was surprised to learn that Uncle Larry had not told them, but he felt the same way we did. It was as if we were trying to preserve Pat's image.

Looking back, I feared that people would judge Pat unfairly when they learned he was sick. I didn't want schizophrenia to become the first thing people thought about when they heard his name. Part of that was my own ignorance about schizophrenia and stereotypes about how it makes people violent.

I also felt that Pat's diagnosis was not mine to disclose, that Pat should tell people himself if that's what he wanted to do. Because Pat hasn't been able to openly say, "Yes, I have schizophrenia," it felt inappropriate to tell someone that he does.

We treat him for it, we agree with his diagnosis, and we maintain his privacy. But to what end? It's not as if he's brought some form of ruin onto himself. Schizophrenia was not his choice. If he had been diagnosed with a brain tumor and was unable to accept that diagnosis, would we also keep that a secret?

When he had trouble performing his duties for work from home because his medication made him very sleepy, Pat's coworkers complained. Dad asked if he wanted to stop working completely, and Pat said yes. We didn't try to encourage or accommodate him, although his illness should have been seen as a disability. If he was a cancer patient on chemotherapy, we would have found a way to help him work, and his coworkers might have been more forgiving of his oversleeping. It was insensitive, but in the moment we didn't recognize it as such.

To this day, Pat does not work. When asked if he considers getting a job, he says he likes to have his time to himself. He spends a great deal of time playing guitar, sometimes recording songs late into the night. He watches a lot of movies and is always asking for recommendations. He seems happy, but it is a solitary life. Everyone needs friends. I often think about what things would have been like if he had never given up his at-home job. If he would have had that modicum of daily social activity, he might be more willing to leave the house today.

Schizophrenia can't be a secret. I've always been a fairly private person, but I've had to let that go. When I talk to close friends about my brother, I never hide his diagnosis. Sometimes they ask questions about schizophrenia, or they just thank me for my honesty. In the beginning, I always expected them to be surprised. I saw a lot of wide eyes back then. But over time that has happened less and less. I don't know if I have been speaking to more worldly people, or if they are less comfortable asking questions, or if they just hide their shock very well. I like to think that they have spoken to other people out there like me and they don't feel like a stranger to severe mental illness.

People with schizophrenia make up about 1 percent of the population. Many people can say they never knew anyone with schizophrenia, but perhaps they knew someone who was a friend or family member of someone with schizophrenia. If we don't let ourselves be known, they'll never realize that. We have a responsibility to advocate for and raise awareness of their illness and their need for adequate care. For years we've feared that an explosive situation might require Pat to be forcibly taken to a mental health facility against his will. We always wanted a better way. Couldn't someone qualified to treat Pat come to him instead? Maybe they could help us convince him to willingly accept their help. How can we ever expect to change these circumstances if we don't educate those around us?

No matter how well Pat is doing, schizophrenia won't let itself be kept in the closet. There are changes in behavior that can be signs of relapse into active-phase psychosis. If we have other people on the lookout for those signs, it makes us better caregivers. We become a network of support for Pat, instead of just three people trying to get through the day.

When the rest of our family learned about Pat's illness, they took it better than expected. Rather than feeling alienated by it, most of them made an effort to understand. They treated him just like the same old Pat. They didn't get their feelings hurt if he wasn't very talkative. His appearance can be a little unsettling if you haven't seen him in a while. He lets his hair and his beard grow long and scraggly. His self-care is lacking, which means greasy hair and unwashed clothes. There's a pungent smell of cigarette smoke when he crosses the room, but it could be worse.

Uncle Larry spends a great deal of time with him. He runs errands for him and checks in on him regularly. He has a level of unmatched patience. His own son passed away in an accident when he was only a teenager. It's given him a great deal of perspective. When it comes to Pat, no matter what happens, he is ours and he is loved. In his own way, Larry makes sure that he always knows that.

In trying to somehow protect Pat, we forget about our own needs. His first symptoms happened right after Hurricane Katrina. None of us ever took the time to heal our wounds after the storm. Mom and Dad worked tirelessly to save the business. I immediately began trying to waylay all of Pat's delusions of persecution, telling myself that nothing was permanently wrong with him. We never stopped to think about how much it hurt to see our beloved hometown in peril. The city was sacked, and those left behind seemed entirely forgotten. Every day radio broadcasts said the same thing: Where is FEMA? Where is the Red Cross? I'll never forget the woman who called the radio station while trapped in her attic. They didn't have anyone they could send to help. I remember a woman in Lakeview, the neighborhood where I went to high school, begging for the water to stop coming. That day we witnessed not only the value of a vibrant old city, the cornerstone of a culture, but the value of human life itself disintegrate right before our eyes. There was no time to weep, to contemplate, or to rail against the people who said we shouldn't rebuild. It was sink or swim.

After Katrina it seemed that anything in the world could happen to us. Everything we thought we understood in our lives was challenged. We knew storms. We grew up with hurricanes. But Katrina still took us by surprise. We knew Pat, but then he got sick, and we didn't seem to know him anymore. He doesn't have the same impressions of Katrina that the rest of our family has. It doesn't loom over him. Perhaps that is a blessing. I often reminisce with my parents about the storm. We refuse to forget all we felt and all the hard living we went through in memory of those who lost everything.

To this day I cannot watch a film or news broadcast about Katrina without great pain in my heart. Homesickness overtakes me. I've had dreams of the storm where I'm in New York and someone tells me the city is gone, New Orleans is wiped from the map. I've dreamed I'm in my old house; the sound of nothing but wind fills my ears; I've lost my parents and I have to go outside in the storm to find them. I've dreamed of a pile slumped in my old yard, something in a sheet or a tarp. I know there's a body underneath, but I won't dare go over and look.

I remember the way it smelled when I went home. It was the smell of mud and spoiled milk, a mixture of all the food that went bad and the reddish mud that washed onto the streets and dried there, cracking in the desperate heat. When I smell something like it, I feel hopeless. Like our lives as they were then, it makes me feel out of control and forgotten. All that anxiety likely contributed to my flying phobia, and it certainly didn't help as Pat's illness set in.

I found that until you begin talking about the diagnosis, it's impossible to accept it. You keep in your heart this dream that it will all just go away. Perhaps the most important reason for talking to others about schizophrenia is the relief it brings. Bottling up the realities we face in caring for someone with mental illness can lead to feeling unhinged ourselves. My outside life is filled with reason. There are no extraordinary delusions, no memory or attention deficits, no hygiene problems or sleepwalking. It's ordinary. Then with Pat, those things are turned upside down. I could carry on keeping them separate, as if I'm leading a double life, or I can intermingle the two, telling Pat about my life out there, and telling others about my brother's illness. Only when I did this did I truly feel free. Like cognitive dissonance, it's troubling to lead two conflicting lifestyles. The reality is that everything can be very normal, and then sometimes it's very messed up. Mental illness is a physical illness, and I won't apologize for the way it might affect my life or the lives of others.

Accepting the diagnosis, accepting my brother, and talking openly about both has brought acceptance to me as well; people can be a lot more understanding than we sometimes give them credit for. And many people offer help and support; others may remain confused or scared, but just talking about mental illness can help people understand it better, watch for signs, and offer help when they can.

Taking on so much responsibility from the very beginning, we as a family forgot one very important part of the equation. We didn't think about ourselves. We felt sadness and stress, but we didn't go looking for a way to make ourselves feel better. Doing that seemed too selfish, too unsupportive of Pat. In the end, everyone has a right to pursue happiness. What good are we to him if we're down? If Mom didn't find satisfaction outside of the home teaching at NAMI, she would feel trapped. Her son would be a burden to her, a ball and chain. That's not fair to anyone. If I hadn't pursued a life in New York, I might have resented Pat eventually.

I finally embraced the idea of my parents dating new people. Who could stand in the way of that bit of happiness given all that they sacrifice in caring for Pat? Taking care of yourself is taking care of your loved ones. It's no different than the pains I took to get my depression under control. Over time, pursuing their own interests, my parents began to brighten up. Each time I speak to them, they are participating in a new social activity, doing lots of volunteer and charity work. They became full-fledged middle-aged divorcees with new hobbies, close friends, and a great deal of support. They have a place to turn when they need help and positive affirmation. They bring that affirmative perspective back home to Pat. When his treatment feels like it is at a standstill, it is still a comfort to feel life and happiness still thriving around him. His support network is full of joy for the taking.

During this time, I became much closer to my mom than I had even been before. When I was a kid, I got the sense that she thought I was too spoiled, too selfish. We were very different kinds of people. She was quiet and reserved, while I was more outspoken and unpredictable.

After NAMI and therapy, she started teaching me a lot about schizophrenia I hadn't considered before. She told me she finally understood Pat's illness through my eyes. She realized I hadn't just lost a brother, but a friend. As she regained her happiness, she also came out of her shell a little. She was more happy-go-lucky and upbeat. We talked more often on the phone, and I started to realize just how much I have in common with my mom. Without her friendship, I know I would have been more worried about Pat's well-being while I was so far away.

17

Coming Together

It took years to find my role in Pat's treatment. Living in another state, I felt utterly ineffectual. If my family needed me, I would have to jump on a plane. Even then, it's not as if I have all the answers. Graduate school taught me that there are many shades to schizophrenia. Talking to a psychopathology professor about Pat's former marijuana use, he asked if he still had an interest in street drugs. "Yeah, he does. When he first got sick, he'd ask if I knew anyone he could buy weed from. If he had the opportunity to smoke it he probably would."

"You know, using is linked to relapse. What's stopping him from going out and getting some weed whenever the mood strikes him?" my professor asked.

I shrugged. "He'd have to call around and interact with people to get it. He doesn't want to do that. He never leaves the house."

"Hmm, how interesting." He was baffled. After years of treating patients with schizophrenia, he had never known someone quite like Pat. Despite the fact that I want my brother's social anxiety to improve, I realize that it has probably kept a lot of other issues contained. I remember friends I met at NAMI talking about their loved one being homeless, leaving home at a young age and moving about constantly, sometimes stealing money from loved ones as well. The fact that Pat has money is scary to some people. They imagine he'll take off some day, motivated by his delusions, and never return. However, he is provided for financially in the form of a trust. It gives him a modicum of independence, but it also sets limits on his spending. He is extremely responsible with his money. Unlike the years before the onset, he saves and buys only what he needs. He never makes large purchases, and he probably doesn't know exactly how much he has saved. If you think about his circumstances, he doesn't have many expenses. Our parents own his home, so he doesn't pay rent or a mortgage, he doesn't drive, and he rarely buys clothing. The majority of his expenses are utilities, groceries, pet supplies, and DVDs (he still loves movies).

Finishing my master's in psychology, I knew a lot more about the origins of schizophrenia, what the drugs do to treat it, and how many things contribute to the outcome. But I didn't know anything more about how to handle it. That was Mom and Dad's domain. While I was away at school, they were face-to-face with the real illness every day. How could I be useful to them? What I failed to see was that I provided advice and support, not just for Pat, but for our parents. Sometimes having a sounding board is all the comfort in the world.

Collectively we began to spot patterns in his illness. His paranoia typically flares up in the fall or early winter. As soon as the weather starts to cool off, Pat withdraws a little more than usual. He has trouble sleeping, and his body language appears anxious or flustered. Sometimes it is accompanied by an actual delusion. For instance, he is very close with his pets. While his dogs have all passed away, he still has one cat. She's not a very friendly pet, but she adores Pat. They are inseparable. In the autumn of 2012, Dad realized that Pat would no longer receive visitors through the front door. They had to enter the house through the garage, lest the cat would run out. While the cat is leery of new people and has never shown an interest in going outside, it was still a serious concern for Pat. Around Thanksgiving, Mom noticed he was even carrying the cat treats around in his pocket, rather than leaving them on the kitchen counter like he used to. It was clear he didn't want to talk about it, but she persisted. Thinking it through, she asked him if he did that because he was worried someone would poison her treats, and he nodded gravely.

Then we have long talks about whether Pat is taking his medication. Dad is usually convinced that he is not, although Mom insists she has seen him take it. I think what is lacking here is our ability to accept the fact that his symptoms may never respond well to drugs. Nonetheless, as February rolls around, his positive symptoms attenuate. He is more relaxed and he sleeps well. His negative symptoms are there, but the delusions are gone until next winter.

It's not that we don't get nervous during these times, but the fact that we see the pattern makes us feel somewhat prepared. Time has also taught me not to expect that certain events in the news or in movies will influence Pat's delusions. I remember hearing in the news several years ago about the discovery of a Russian spy ring in the United States. It led to a lot of jokes from comedians and TV personalities poking fun, saying how these spies apparently never got word that the Cold War had ended. It wasn't so funny to me. I immediately thought, "Oh, great. I wonder how Pat will process this." At the time he was delusional, off medication and refusing to bathe because he felt there was a camera in the showerhead. He watched television regularly and certainly heard about the spy ring on the news, but he had no reaction. It didn't interest him or play into his delusions about being spied on himself.

Delusions aren't so simple. I never know how his paranoia will manifest itself. Even if something seems to fit well into a persecutory delusion, it doesn't mean Pat will take the bait, so to speak. I've seen him find confirmation of his suspicions in the most innocuous things. A simple noise, whether it's the settling of the house at night or maybe the cat walking down the hallway, could confirm to him that people are coming into the house when he's in bed. A stray wire in an old junk drawer or a battery that has fallen on the floor in the garage are confirmation that someone has been installing cameras or listening devices in the house. As I've said before, he doesn't require a reason for being watched. He claims he wants to know who is keeping him under surveillance and why, but he doesn't venture a guess.

Accepting how unpredictable the delusions are was a comfort to me. My heart doesn't sink every time I hear about spies, stalkers, wiretaps, hidden cameras, or some other conspiracy. Finally I don't tense up when watching the news. His paranoia is not something anyone can control. We just have to face it as it comes, think quickly on our feet, and try to identify with his delusions rather than dismiss them out of hand. There is no expert way of confronting delusions, but I have learned not to be pragmatic and try to reason with him. Instead, we all try to sympathize with his concerns and give him alternative explanations for his suspicions. We sit side by side and try to solve the problem. Being confrontational or didactic isn't helpful, and it usually leads to him no longer wanting to communicate or share his concerns.

While most of the family still doesn't play an active role in Pat's life, each of us who does has a part to play, and it isn't a far cry from how it used to be. We were always supportive. The burden of communication falls more heavily on our shoulders. While he keeps to himself and doesn't volunteer much in a conversation, we've grown accustomed to it. We just persevere. We encourage him to pursue new hobbies, even if he doesn't stick with them. Dad helped him set up an entire workout room, although he doesn't exercise now. Mom has to remind him to tidy the house, clean the litter box, and bathe. Larry reminds him of things he might need, groceries that he's forgotten to ask for.

In 2012, Pat began taking a new antipsychotic. We were excited about it because it was different from the daily pills he had taken in the past. This drug is a long-term injection that is given to him once a month. A registered nurse comes to his home to administer it. Just his willingness to have a stranger come into his home, his willingness in general to receive guests, is proof of real compromise on his part. I know the thought of it made him anxious. After a year, his response to the drug is about the same as it has been with other drugs. He doesn't have any positive symptoms other than a winter flare-up. We consider this to be baseline and think he would be making more progress with the addition of cognitive behavioral therapy. There is still a lack of hygiene, and he has to be reminded to bathe. He still doesn't leave the house, but everyone continues to run his errands. Perhaps given some incremental changes, we will see more social recovery. That, however, is not under my control.

Mom moved out of her home and back to her hometown to care for her elderly mother. Pat now lives there on his own. He cooks for himself and cleans up after himself. He cares for his cat. He's even moved some furniture around to suit his own tastes. Dad's house is just half an hour away, and Uncle Larry stops by nearly every day. Mom makes regular visits to stay with him. Most of her time there is spent helping Pat clean the house. He sees his psychiatrist once a month, but there are times when he cancels these appointments. Again, this probably has something to do with his social anxiety. He would prefer having someone accompany him when he has to go out, but there is not always someone available to go with him.

At least now there is no question of whether he is taking his medication. I can finally separate the behaviors that are symptomatic of schizophrenia and the quirks that are just Pat being Pat. Social anxiety or living like a hermit are not symptomatic. Many people with schizophrenia partake in day-to-day activities like grocery shopping, driving, going to the pharmacy, visiting relatives, and so forth. Pat's refusal to leave the house is accommodated when others bring him everything he needs. A step in the right direction would be for people to ask him to at least come with them when they run his errands. Over time, after being exposed to new places full of strangers and potential social interactions, he might take the initiative to run his errands himself. I am convinced that this would be the first step in his social and occupational recovery. Implementing these changes, however, falls on Dad's shoulders. It's very difficult to give up control and then sometimes need to take it back. Pat needs his space and room to grow, but at the same time he is stubborn and in need of incentives to accept responsibility.

Routines are a large part of recovery in schizophrenia. A predictable schedule can be comforting. It also helps to combat the negative symptoms of memory and motivation problems. It may not occur to schizophrenics to wash and fold their laundry, but if it is a regularly scheduled activity, they have a better chance of remembering. In Pat's case, his routines are the first thing to change when he begins to relapse. He doesn't get up at the usual hour, he has trouble getting to bed, and he even forgets something he normally does every day.

He eats at the same time every day. He drinks beer on a nightly basis, but he is careful not to drink too much. When he does have a beer, he becomes more talkative and comes out of his bedroom. He'll actually stand in the kitchen and talk with me or even sit down in the living room. On several occasions when he has been stressed, for instance when one of his dogs passed away, he might drink a little more than usual. Of course, Dr. Russell has prescribed antianxiety medicine for stressful times, but Pat doesn't like how groggy it makes him feel. "Beer relaxes me," he says. "Those drugs just knock me out."

That is why our parents compromise on his drinking. We would prefer that he didn't drink at all. An alcohol interaction with his medication can cause increased drowsiness, impaired judgment, and poor psychomotor skills. Alcohol does have a history of affecting his sleep. It can make him restless and even cause him to sleepwalk. On the other hand, his alcohol is supplied for him. He gets a certain amount of beer per week, and he has to ration that out. It keeps his consumption under control. He has maybe two or three beers a night over the course of several hours. Also, since he has been on the long-term injection, he rarely sleepwalks. I believe he has taken care to strike a balance.

After about six months on the injection, Pat started to talk more often about his personal history. He volunteers information about his life, showing not only improved memory but also a personal frame of reference in order to relate to other people.

At Thanksgiving dinner, when my aunt complained about her recent weight gain, he pointed out that it followed a fall in which she broke her arm. "That's when I started having trouble with my weight. I was in seventh grade when I broke my arm playing basketball." He showed her the long scar down his arm. "I had to quit the tennis team. All of a sudden I put on a lot of weight, and it took forever to lose it."

I stood there agape. I knew something significant had changed. The fact that he was opening up and talking about himself was shocking. Part of me worried that something was wrong, but I shook it off. It was the return of self-awareness, of identity talk. I basked in it. We reminisced all evening.

The next month he wanted to set up his garage as a workout room, complete with air-conditioning unit and rubber mats. Dad helped him move the workout equipment in there and even helped him wire up a TV. Pat never stuck to using it, though. I felt bad for Dad going to all that trouble, but I'm still happy Pat *wanted* to do it to begin with, so rarely is he motivated to make big changes to his routine or his living space. Exercise is also self-improvement, something he hasn't shown any interest in since his diagnosis.

But if there's a new level of self-awareness, then doesn't he have questions about his therapy? He has still never recognized his illness or had any psychoeducation outside of what Dr. Russell tells him about the medication side effects. It was time to see how much he knew, how much he recognized. That's when Mom asked him what he thought about his therapy one day as they left Dr. Russell's office. "Do you understand why you see a psychiatrist, why you take medication?"

"Yeah, sure," he said vaguely.

"How do you feel knowing that you've been diagnosed with schizophrenia?" she asked more specifically.

"Look, Mom, I know I'm weird. I understand that I need help."

Satisfied, she left it at that.

There were more improvements to follow. Once, Pat had been highly interested in politics, even making a brief foray into graduate study in political science. After his diagnosis in 2006, he no longer voted. In 2012, not only did he vote in the presidential election, but he even made a generous campaign donation. He texted me and told me to go vote. Sometimes he would text me to tell me he liked a particular movie or a new album that just came out. One night he messaged me a picture of his cat. She was sprawled out on her back looking fat and comfy. His message was simply, "Who's the best cat in the world?"

There are times when Pat can still be very obstinate and set in his ways, not wanting to do anything new. Living in a three-bedroom house by himself requires plenty of upkeep. He cleans up here and there, but spring cleaning is never on his agenda. A layer of dust coats baseboards and rarely used shelves. Dust bunnies hide under the furniture and behind doors. Mom has to strike a deal with him to get him to do these more intensive tasks. It's a fairly ingenious method. If Pat wants her to pick him up some cigarettes, then he has to complete a few goals like sweeping up, taking a bath, and washing his clothes. He always agrees, but he often has trouble with execution. The token phrase is, "We had an agreement, Pat, and you broke it." Usually by the next day he's completed all his goals. In a way, it's helped Pat to accept the fact that relationships are symbiotic. You have to mean what you say and hold up your half of the bargain.

His best friend growing up went to school out of state. Newlyweds, he and his wife recently had a baby boy. Since he hadn't shown much interest before, I was surprised at how tickled it made Pat. The baby was born near his birthday, and he thought that was pretty great. He still hasn't reached out to his old friends, but I understand it's complicated. At times when he was actively psychotic, he had called them, made accusations, and probably scared them. While everyone wants to talk to him, I think Pat is the one mired in guilt and afraid to make contact. I'm sure he wouldn't want to explain to his old friends that he doesn't leave home or have a career. As I told him, one step at a time.

It wasn't very long until I got my first e-mail from Pat in six years. Even better was what it contained. The subject was "One of my songs," and the message read only, "Give it a chance." He attached a music file, a song he wrote on the guitar and recorded. He wanted to know what I thought. Nothing could have prepared me for hitting play. It wasn't different, disjointed, simplified, or unmelodic. It was the same as any song he had written before his illness. All of his technical skill and writing ability was intact. It was like hearing Pat's voice again for the first time in six years. His real voice was talking to me. The style sounded like him. The recording was clean; he had spent a lot of time working on it. There was even a happy, jaunty interlude a few minutes in.

I told him it was great; then I cried like a baby. He e-mailed me again asking for more feedback.

After that, my whole day became a surreal reverie. What's going on? How could this be? We've never had him back again so whole. It was brilliant and terrifying all at once. You want to wrap yourself up in your glee, and then you fear you'll lose it again.

I knew that he wasn't entirely recovered, perfectly healthy, or back to his old self. He still has breakthrough symptoms on his medication, hygiene problems, and delusional thinking. Dr. Russell even admits that for all the drugs they've tried, Pat may never be responsive to antipsychotic drugs. Refractory schizophrenia, it's called, and an estimated 30 percent of people with schizophrenia have this kind.[1] There may truly be no end in sight for any of his symptoms.

But when I listened to that song, it sounded like any song that the healthy Pat would have written before the onset of his schizophrenia. It gave me hope that while he may never be the same man he was, some things weren't taken away from him. He has creative ideas, he enjoys making music, and he uses that outlet to find a modicum of satisfaction.

Even now, when I listen to that song, I am a teenager again. I swim in our kidney-shaped pool and sneak out my window at night to smoke cigarettes. I can smell the chlorine. I sleep all day and watch movies with him on Friday nights. We always get the same pizza, pepperoni with extra cheese. I'm a college student living off of Rally's french fries. My hair is every color. I live with my brother in a house in New Orleans. He's a homebody, and he likes me to bring him frozen coffees when I go out. It may sound bittersweet, but being transported back to a healthier time feels good. I didn't think it was possible anymore.

Sometimes I wonder, "How could anything in this world be too hard for me, if Pat can do all this?" It inspires me.

Above all else, listening to the music I felt something that surprised me, something that I didn't know was dangling over my head all these years. For the first time since 2007, I felt like I was no longer alone in the world.

Is he satisfied in his life? He seems to be. And because of that we ought to be satisfied too. Will he ever work again? Will he go back to school? Will he ever answer e-mails or phone calls from his old college buddies? I can't know that. I try not to set my heart on what could be and try to embrace what is.

He knows that our parents and I will always be there for him and that he can talk to us via phone or e-mail whenever he pleases. He reaches out when he needs us and appreciates us when we take an active part in his treatment. Support and patience are the greatest things we can offer him. Mom, Dad, and I have been rewarded for hanging in there, and we will continue to do so.

Part 4

STEPS TOWARD RECOVERY

18

Fighting Stigma

The stigmatization of mental illness is a steadfast barrier to recovery. Imagine having an incurable disease that makes people fearful and distrustful of you rather than sympathetic. The most common mistake is assuming that mental illness is not physical, the implication being that the illness is under the control of the afflicted. Health insurance does not cover many aspects of treatment, likely because of the idea that mental health is voluntary. There's also the fact that schizophrenia is incurable. The insurance company imagines a whole lifetime of relapse and hospitalization ahead of Pat. It's not a very helpful outlook.

In a way it's true. Treatment of schizophrenia requires more than just drugs. It's an ongoing process that requires so much work on the part of the afflicted that it's hardly even fair. Pat looks well. He's not wasting away in a hospital bed. He is able bodied. For the most part, he has all his wits about him. Because of that, people fail to be sensitive to his condition. Rarely is he cut any slack. I've heard people call his lifestyle lazy. His former coworkers were critical of how much he slept. They seem to know that sometimes he has delusions, but they can't wrap their head around the negative symptoms that affect his memory, attention, and social behavior. They assume his lack of hygiene, monosyllabic speech, lack of facial expression, low motivation (avolition), inability to experience pleasure (anhedonia), and lack of contributing to a conversation (alogia) are voluntary. I joked with Pat recently that I would make him a T-shirt that read, "I'm not awkward. I have schizophrenia."

The fact is that many people don't understand what schizophrenia is. Many would dismiss psychoeducation out of hand, saying, "I know what schizophrenia is. That's when someone is totally insane." Some people think schizophrenia has something to do with "split personality," mistaking it for the personality disorder otherwise known as dissociative identity disorder (DID). People with schizophrenia do not have multiple personalities.

People often believe that schizophrenia follows an easily recognizable psychotic break that leads to hospitalization and diagnosis. They imagine the person "snapped" and was found sitting in their kitchen mumbling quietly, as if in a trance. This fails to take into account an insidious onset like Pat's. It also suggests that in a particular moment the person lost his grip on reality. Some event set it off. We would all love to put our finger on one thing that led to schizophrenia. Of course it's not that simple.

People don't know the battle inside. They don't realize what fear does to someone with schizophrenia, how the afflicted buy into the stigma, making it hard to help them. The average person probably gets the majority of their information about schizophrenia from television and movies. Unfortunately when schizophrenia makes headlines it is in association with an extraordinary, violent, criminal act. This is the only exposure the illness gets, contributing to the idea that schizophrenics are violent, dangerous individuals. It can be hard for schizophrenics to find housing and work because of this. In reality, people with schizophrenia are more likely to hurt themselves than someone else. Once you consider the fear and trepidation they feel, striking out seems understandable.

Violent outbursts usually occur at home. It's caregivers like us who are most likely to be affected. Twentieth-century deinstitutionalization was a response to lawsuits claiming that being institutionalized against one's will violated people's civil rights. Mental health facilities that were poorly run helped to make the case that hospitals didn't know what was best for these individuals. What we often don't think about is where these people in need of critical care went. They no longer had regular therapy, there was no socio-occupational safety net, and they did not have to take medication. A great deal of research since then has shown that schizophrenia is more common among homeless people than in the population at large.[1] I found it interesting that many people think they've never met a schizophrenic because they are hospitalized somewhere, even after deinstitutionalization. In reality, they probably saw a schizophrenic in the subway that very morning and didn't realize it.

In 2011, twenty-two-year-old Jared Lee Loughner was arrested for shooting Representative Gabrielle Giffords and eighteen others in a supermarket parking lot in Tucson, Arizona. After his arrest, Loughner was diagnosed with schizophrenia. There was a public outcry. People wanted to know if there were warning signs and if someone, especially his parents, should have intervened before the shooting. The problem is that the public assumed two things: that violence is inherent in schizophrenia and that there is something we can do to control or contain a person with mental illness. During the trial, a court order was issued to forcibly medicate Loughner at a nonmedical correctional facility.[2] It seems they wanted to make Loughner well so that he could take responsibility for something he did while psychotic and not in his right mind.

Making a medical intervention after the fact cannot undo the damage that was done. Making him well in order to stand trial flies in the face of reason. If he could not be involuntarily medicated before he committed a heinous crime, why should he be medicated afterward? It could be viewed as a form of punishment to make him understand the difference between real and unreal, to make him possibly come to realize what a terrible thing he has done. Families like mine felt that if this could happen to Loughner, it could happen to our loved ones too.

Loughner's case is a perfect example of how our hands are tied until our loved ones hurt themselves or others. The lack of adequate mental health care in America makes it difficult to treat the mentally ill before something terrible happens—before a suicide, or a violent outburst, or a psychotic break that leads someone to live on the streets.

Families are often left with the burden of dealing with the severely mentally ill, those who are in the most danger of hurting themselves or others. And many families don't have the resources or the education to know if a family member has an illness or to treat it.

The association between mental illness and violence is so steeped in our national culture that mass shootings immediately make people start talking about mental health. When the public begins to weigh in on the state of mental health in our country, all I want them to do is take an active concern in the accessibility of care for mental health patients. Given the circumstances, let's take steps to make it more likely that people will get help than that they will hurt themselves or others. Adequate affordable health care would be a start. Of course there is no promise that people with schizophrenia would seek treatment. Perhaps they would if there were incentives in place for them to do so.

Forcibly medicating someone with schizophrenia is considered a civil rights violation, unless it's court ordered and distributed in a prison, sometimes not even by a qualified health-care provider.[3]

When Mom learned how many patients in her NAMI class had been arrested, she was flabbergasted. Many of them had recently been to the emergency room with positive symptoms but were released because doctors had no reason to believe they were a danger to themselves or others. One man said the first time his son ever took antipsychotic medication was when it was forcibly given to him while incarcerated for throwing a brick through a woman's garage.

The teacher that Mom assisted had a teenage daughter who, at fifteen, attempted suicide twice, both times right after being released from the hospital. It broke Mom's heart to hear that. "I wish there were laws protecting Pat's right to be healthy, rather than laws protecting his right to be insane," she said.

When we imagine institutionalized people with mental illness, it's easy to think about the lives they left behind. What's missing from the conversation is what became of them afterward. No one who supported deinstitutionalization thought freedom was a cure of some sort. We felt that institutionalization was a way of locking the mentally ill away and forgetting about them, but once they were free they were still forgotten. Without adequate community-based treatment, we didn't give them anything to replace the care and safety they'd once had institutionally. Their quality of life is now their own responsibility. Lucky ones were taken in and cared for by family and loved ones. For some, the financial burden of doing that was too much to handle. For others, many others perhaps, even when shelter and care are offered by family or friends, getting help can be difficult.

The misconception of schizophrenia is readily apparent in film. There's always a trick in movies. The schizophrenic realizes that he's the man who killed his wife. The schizophrenic realizes that she isn't actually being stalked, that she has in fact been stalking herself. Of course, this doesn't make sense.

This idea of "losing time" while another personality takes over your body is not schizophrenia. It's dissociative identity disorder, more commonly known as multiple personality disorder. Furthermore, when a schizophrenic realizes they were wrong about something, that there was no danger or persecution all along, that doesn't make them suddenly think, "Oh, I'm schizophrenic. Someone, quick, give me some Thorazine. Someone make me an appointment with a psychologist. I promise to consider your feedback and never take my perception of reality for granted again."

In movies, they still lock up schizophrenics. Now they show them in hospitals for the criminally insane who have committed acts so unspeakable they trump every "sane" serial killer in history. There is no responsibility taken for the way these depictions stigmatize mental illness because they are works of fiction. But schizophrenia is not fiction. It's not a fantasy like vampires, werewolves, and other movie monsters. Stigma disenfranchises the mentally ill and stands squarely in the way of recovery. Pat has a right to lead a normal and fulfilling life just like anyone else.

I take exception whenever people say something ill informed about mental illness. Nothing could have prepared me for the stigma I found in school during my graduate study in psychology. Other master's students would say remarkably insensitive things about the mentally ill. One student told me that she turned down an externship to work at an outpatient facility treating people diagnosed with schizophrenia.

"Why? Was it unpaid?" I asked.

"No, it's just dangerous. They don't have a guard on duty there."

I sat there a moment, staring at my desk and fuming. I couldn't think of a single time I had heard of a therapist attacked by a schizophrenic at any of our externship facilities.

"What?" she asked.

"If they're coming to outpatient care," I said calmly, "they're medicated. It's unlikely that it's dangerous."

"How do you know that?"

"Well, if you think about it at all, they probably won't show up to outpatient care if they went off their meds. If they're psychotic, that facility is the last place they'd want to be." I picked up my things, ready to leave the classroom.

"What? What did I say?"

"Just think next time before you speak." I stormed off.

I had no patience for ignorance in grad school. Many of those students hoped to one day treat people like Pat. In her defense, the student did not know that my brother has schizophrenia. She was, however, a PhD student on her way to becoming a licensed clinical psychologist.

Some of my classmates knew of Pat's diagnosis, and they were always in tune with me when schizophrenia came up in lectures. One day a classmate was talking about the social work she had done at a clinic in Manhattan that served people with severe mental illness living in halfway homes. She met so many patients with schizophrenia that she felt she was an authority. "It's so sad, you guys. All of them have such terrible family histories. The things they've seen—all of them. It's just so dysfunctional and abusive."

A close friend of mine interrupted her. Turning to me, she said, "Wow, Sarah, how does it make you feel to hear someone talk about your brother like that?"

"It makes me sad." I said. I could feel the whole class holding its breath.

"Oh," the other student said, "I didn't realize—"

"There's nothing particularly menacing about my family. We weren't beaten or neglected or starved or otherwise. Our home life wasn't perfect, no one's is, and I turned out healthy."

"I'm only talking about my own experience."

"Maybe you should preface your comments with that next time," my friend told her. The class let out a collective breath, and we continued with our roundtable discussion on dual diagnosis.

Having pretty much announced to the class that I was the sister of a schizophrenic left me feeling a little resentful. Instead of asking me questions about him, the disease, or his treatment history, people more often just told me they were sorry, as if I deserved condolences.

On another occasion the same classmate was talking about how poor her patients' hygiene was, how one smelled so bad that she had to suspend the intake interview. I didn't argue with her then. Not every schizophrenic has hygiene problems. More than anything, the issue seems to be that they just don't think about practicing hygiene. While I get up every morning, take a shower, brush my teeth, and comb my hair, Pat doesn't think to do that. Of course, I think it's easier for him to forget about self-care because he has had delusions about the bathroom. In the past he had suspicions that there were spy cameras in the bathroom, but since then he has said that's no longer a concern.

As of now, he doesn't really consider himself to be dirty if he doesn't smell. When medication didn't improve his lack of hygiene, I wondered if something was wrong. Shouldn't the medication fix that? Apparently not. My friend Steve, whom I met through blogging about schizophrenia, was diagnosed with schizophrenia at age nineteen. He is medicated and has always had trouble with self-care. "I wake up one day and realize I haven't bathed in so long I can't even remember the last time. I'm ashamed of it," he told me.

"Do you dislike being in the bathroom?" I asked him.

"There was one time in the shower, I thought I heard my professor describing everything I was doing."

"Is that when the hygiene problem started?"

"I have to tell you, I have no idea whatsoever if that's when it started. I do know that it's easier to make it part of my routine when someone else is doing it. You know, I get up with my wife, and she showers, so I would shower afterward to follow her example."

Pat lives alone and doesn't get up until noon. There isn't a prime example of a routine at his fingertips. I did feel better knowing it was an issue for other medicated schizophrenics.

"I still don't really like it, though," Steve said.

I wondered about it for a moment and said, "You know, I guess I just never think about bathing. I just do it, like I'm on autopilot."

Most people I talk to about schizophrenia don't realize that poor hygiene is a negative symptom. You might not connect self-care to symptomatology at all, especially if you're thinking about a homeless person with schizophrenia. Then lack of hygiene would seem simply circumstantial.

When I think about my routine in the bathroom, I understand how it can become a place of contention. Getting into the shower or bath requires disrobing. Nakedness is a particularly vulnerable state. If your thoughts are wrapped up in feelings of persecution or you hear persecutory voices in your head, being nude can be very uncomfortable. Self-care also isn't very exciting. Brushing one's teeth is not a very fun or stimulating task in itself. Washing one's hair and putting on cologne may not seem important to some people. I always told myself that Pat was just concerned with other things than hygiene, and I think that is more than likely true.

Often when we talk about stigma, we don't think about how the stigmatization surrounding schizophrenia makes it hard for the schizophrenic to accept the diagnosis. Shortly after he stopped taking his medication in 2008, Pat called me to confront me about some of his suspicions. I asked if he thought perhaps his mounting anxiety had anything to do with his medication noncompliance.

"What does that have to do with it?" he asked.

"Perhaps there is a pattern here," I said. "Maybe the schizophrenia is flaring up because you suddenly stopped taking your medicine."

"Schizophrenia?"

"Pat, you were diagnosed with schizophrenia by Dr. Hollis at the end of 2006."

"Sarah, if I had schizophrenia, I'd be locked in a padded cell somewhere. I'd be in a hospital, in a straitjacket."

"That's not true," I said, stunned to hear the stigma I thought I was fighting coming out of my brother's mouth. "People with schizophrenia can enter therapy, take medication, and live perfectly normal lives. Schizophrenics can have jobs and spouses and families."

He had stopped listening to me. I'm sure he didn't believe me. It is still my hope that one day he will attend group therapy. I believe that meeting others with the same condition would give him a great deal of perspective. I think he would be inspired.

It is incredible to think how differently things would be if he had been diagnosed with another condition. Pat couldn't accept schizophrenia, but there was a time when he told me he thought he had bipolar disorder. That was a more acceptable diagnosis to him. After that, he even considered Asperger syndrome—high-functioning autism—as an explanation for his high intelligence and difficulty socializing. Even Asperger's was more acceptable than schizophrenia. At the same time, he was able to admit that his problems were not under his control. That has probably helped us a great deal.

There were times when even our family fell prey to stigma. A fund was set up to aid those who were diagnosed with mental illness after Hurricane Katrina. Pat's therapist and a nurse who worked for him both explained the process to Mom for filing a claim on Pat's behalf. The window for filing for aid closed in 2008. We never filed a claim. Our parents felt it was inappropriate. They could provide for Pat themselves. However, I think their decision was guided more by their denial and hope that Pat would be fine, and also by their desire not to appear needy. If they had considered the fact that he would not be able to work one day, perhaps they would have made a different decision. It's unfortunate that he was off his medication and delusional in 2008 because I can only wonder if he would have wanted to file a claim himself. The choice ultimately should have been his.

Our initial compulsion to keep the diagnosis to ourselves also had its root in stigma. Thinking about it now reminds me of families in the early nineteenth century. People with mental illness were sent away to mental institutions, hidden away from the rest of society. They might be hospitalized hundreds of miles from home, even in another state. There was no hope of them being rehabilitated and leaving the hospital. Cordoned off so that the world at large didn't have to see or worry about them, some were forsaken by their relatives like a dark family secret. People didn't want it to get out that a relative "had gone mad" less it change their prospects of marrying or getting a job.

I know we didn't want to secrete away Pat's illness, but there was no easy way to let everyone know what was happening and make sure they understood it all. It was such a big change from how things used to be that it seemed impossible to tell someone about it without them thinking I was the one who was insane. Oddly enough, other people seemed to have an easier time accepting it than I did.

Today, as a family, we own schizophrenia. We bust stigma, avoid falling into stereotypical thinking, and remain hopeful no matter what we see on TV or in the movies. We are brave in the face of flare-ups. We have our peeves and quirks. For instance, I often abbreviate schizophrenia by writing "SZ." Rarely do people not affected by the illness know what I mean.

When talking about Pat, our family uses the term "schizophrenic" rather than broader, all-encompassing terms like "mentally ill" or "mental health consumer." It's important to us that people know the particular illness. Obscuring his diagnosis leads people to believe that schizophrenia is too rare to affect anyone they know.

Mom doesn't like when people use the term "schizophrenic" to describe something that doesn't make sense, is disjointed, or doesn't follow suit. It's become a popular way of critiquing films, books, or performances. It's used in a dismissive way, and that's the last thing we want associated with schizophrenia. Pat is a musician, and when he composes a song on the guitar there is nothing *schizophrenic* about it.

After the shooting at Sandy Hook Elementary School in Newtown, Connecticut, someone asked Mom casually if Pat had experience with guns. Although it's tiresome hearing Pat lumped in with every "crazy" person in the news, we try to answer questions without getting angry. Of course, that was particularly hard for me when I was talking to future clinical psychologists. But if a person seems honestly concerned and genuinely unaware that the question could be inflammatory, we answer them honestly.

I don't have concerns that my brother will do something violent. I'm more concerned that someone will call me one day to tell me he has taken off and they don't know where he is. I have no reason to believe he would do this other than all the stories I've heard from other families about their loved one's running away. I read a story once about a schizophrenic who would sleepwalk at night. They found him frozen to death on a bench across the street from his house. Thankfully Pat sets a very loud burglar alarm and deadbolts his doors at night.

The prevalence of suicide is something left out of the movies. Suicide is a major cause of death in schizophrenia. Suicide has been estimated to account for 5 to 13 percent of deaths in schizophrenia patients.[4] Depression is so high there is a diagnostic disorder called postpsychotic depressive disorder. This is a condition that may occur during the residual phase of schizophrenia, when positive symptoms have attenuated and the patient enters a period of depression. Once their positive symptoms are gone, awareness of the time they have lost to active psychosis, the relationships that have changed, or the job they might have lost is too hard to bear.

Certain risk factors contribute to postpsychotic depressive disorder and coincidentally to suicide in schizophrenia. These include having had a high level of success before the onset of schizophrenia or before their last psychotic episode, living alone, having few social supports, experiencing relapse despite medication compliance, having a long list of hospitalizations, and having had an insidious (slow) onset. Many of these things are true of Pat's illness. The best we can do is remain vigilant and keep communication open.

In the end, every time I hear or see something disparaging or uninformed about schizophrenia, it can feel like a setback. I begin to feel like recovery is that much further away from us. Meeting other people who get amped up about beating mental illness stigma was comforting for me. The National Alliance on Mental Illness has 5K walks in every state to raise funds that support mental health and fight stigma. For me it has been a wonderful experience. Sometimes group meetings at NAMI can be heavy, serious, and even harrowing. But at a walk you can be sure there will be nothing but smiling faces. Going out to South Street Seaport in Manhattan on a Saturday morning with a large group of caregivers, mental health practitioners, and the families and friends of the mentally ill, I feel at home. Warming up with happy, energetic people in their brightly colored shirts with team names like "Stigma Police" on their backs makes me feel humble and thankful every time.

Facing the Future

Although the development of schizophrenia is considered to be the product of genes and environment, it does often run in families. While Pat's was the first diagnosis in our family, there could be more in the future. In this way, schizophrenia leaves an indelible mark. One diagnosis could mean a Pandora's box of diagnoses.

I have a 9 percent chance of developing the illness by age thirty-five. If I have children with someone with no family history of schizophrenia, our child's chances of developing schizophrenia are only 3 percent.[1] While genes do not take full responsibility for the development of schizophrenia, the data show that the more relatives, especially first-degree relatives, one has with schizophrenia, the more likely one is to develop the illness too. Taken at face value, my odds are very good. On the other hand, I want to feel prepared for the possibility. I never want to be taken by surprise by schizophrenia again.

Women tend to develop schizophrenia later in life than males. Considering how much I have grown in the last six years and how much I know about schizophrenia, I can't imagine having the illness myself. I've always needed a lot of feedback from people around me to reassure me. Then again, so did Pat. I've considered the ways in which we are similar now: anxious, uncomfortable in social situations, introverted, and preferring solitary hobbies. I cringe when I hear my neighbors in the hallway, hoping they won't knock on my door.

I close my drapes if someone across the street has their window open or is out on their balcony. But I don't shy away from social interaction. I speak to strangers in elevators, filling awkward silence with idle chitchat. I consider a conversation a success if I can make a person I just met chuckle. It's a little pick-me-up that makes me look forward to spontaneous meetings.

I know Pat wouldn't enjoy running into people while he's checking his mail or putting out his garbage. We did have more in common when we were younger. I didn't like meeting new people, either. Parties were full of trepidation. I would cling to one person all night or just bail at the last minute before the party. If a neighbor rang my doorbell, I probably acted as if I wasn't home. I most certainly never thought to go over to their house to say hello or borrow something. Self-reliance is an important skill, but it's very lonely.

I've matured out of certain habits. I'm not set in my ways or easily given to feeling annoyed or angry. I don't worry about what other people are thinking and rarely ever feel like people are staring when I walk down the subway platform. Exposure to social situations on a regular basis helped me to be more calm and reasonable. Making new friends requires a great deal of perspective taking and sympathizing. You have to meet people halfway. You can't make friends on just your own terms. I think wrapping his head around that would be a hurdle for Pat. On the other hand, he would say he's not interested in making friends anyway.

I consider myself to be a very self-aware person. I meditate. I keep a journal, consider my shortcomings, think about how I might have handled something better, and try to find ways to improve myself incrementally. Once Dr. Little helped me get through my flying phobia, I felt like I could change anything. I'm not crazy about self-help books, but when I can't find a new way of looking at something I'll visit a bookshop and comb through the stacks. I try to be aware of the ways my anxiety holds me back from doing the things I want or being the person I want to be.

Of course, all this is easier said than done. The way we interact with the world around us is largely habitual. When you're not aware of what you're doing, how you're reacting to something, it's difficult to change that behavior and incorporate something new. I like to think of myself as a work in progress, and the work will probably never be complete. This allows me to take my time, consider new issues as they come, and stop beating myself up for not being perfect right now.

When I think about my approach, it doesn't jibe with schizophrenia. Perhaps I could still descend into it and everything about me would change. During the onset of schizophrenia, there is a lack of self-awareness. It's unlikely a person will realize on their own that their concerns aren't real and head over to an emergency room asking for psychiatric help. If they realize a change in their senses, they don't associate those changes with the onset of an illness. And how could they? Who thinks that one day, amid adulthood, they would succumb to an illness that would change everything about their personality?

Considering the fact that I could become sick without realizing it, I take precautions. I told my boyfriend, Gavin, about some warning signs to look for: social withdrawal, sleep problems, stopping hobbies, and so forth. He has the phone number for the Psychiatry Department at Columbia University in the event that I start showing symptoms and need an evaluation. Columbia was doing a study on the onset of schizophrenia in people with first-degree relatives that have the illness. Years later, I have no idea if they are still doing this research. In fact, we don't want to know. We put our fears behind us that I would get sick too. Having a plan for something like that is impossible and unhelpful. Who knows how the illness would manifest itself. Better to cross that bridge when we come to it, if we ever come to it.

The idea that I could become sick is a possibility that I rarely even think about now, until something strange happens. Say I have a day where I'm constantly looking over my shoulder because I think I hear someone behind me. Maybe I feel like people on the subway are looking at me and judging me. Maybe I think the clerk at the store smiled because my hair looks messy. When these things happen, I tell myself I need to get out more. I'm imagining these things because I've been too isolated at home. Sure enough, once I go out more, I don't have days like this.

Some days I have trouble shaking the feeling that someone is standing behind me or watching me from the next room. It's as if everything out of the corner of my eye looks like a person. When I look, nothing is there. Maybe my hair was just in my face. It could very well be that scary movie I watched recently or the horror novel I read last month. Thinking about scary things gives anyone the creeps. Who knows? The sheer fact that I acknowledge these things makes me feel secure about myself.

It gets stranger. There are mornings before I'm fully awake, lying there on the brink of consciousness, thinking about snoozing my alarm, when my phonological loop gets very pliable. Remember what I said earlier about the phonological loop? The articulatory or phonological loop is part of working memory. It's that part of your memory store that houses snippets of what you hear for a moment. This is what you're using while your professor talks and you feverishly try to scribble down what she says. It's postulated by neurologists that hearing voices in one's head could be the result of a faulty phonological loop. The patient can't tell the different between real sound and the sounds generated or regenerated in their mind. I've never heard voices in my head, but I have sleepily heard things I've imagined. In that place between being asleep and awake, I feel like I can really hear anything I bring to mind. If I imagine a foghorn, I hear it in my ear, and startle fully awake. I might imagine a word, and then hear someone saying that word clearly. Then I'll sit up tensely, checking that the room is empty.

My alarm is set to play the sound of birds chirping. I swear that when I turn it off, I lie in bed, still hearing their song. I've even checked to see if there were any birds outside.

It only happens in the morning, during shallow sleep, never at night. This didn't start happening until a few years ago. I was about twenty-seven years old the first time it happened. At first it made me feel crazy. I talked to Gavin about it nervously, afraid he would think it was scary. He said a lot of people experience funny things when they're half awake. Over time I grew accustomed to this "sound phenomenon" happening, and now it no longer frightens me. On mornings when it happens, I think to myself, "Well, there it is again."

I go to bed some nights with jittery hands, arms, legs, and feet. It's like there is a current of electricity running through my limbs. I can't lie still. Every position makes me want to reposition myself. I learned in graduate school that dropping off to sleep requires an increase of serotonin and decrease of dopamine in the brain. I lie there thinking I'm full of dopamine. Serotonin isn't doing its job like it did for my boyfriend beside me. It won't rise and let me drift off to sleep. Why can't I sleep? What's going to happen next? It doesn't help that I start thinking about it. It sends my mind racing, and that surely won't help me get to sleep.

As for raising a family and worrying about my children developing schizophrenia, my old psychologist Dr. Little recommended I see a genetic counselor before starting a family. It seemed alarmist to me. My children's chances of getting schizophrenia are only 3 percent. I've been dating the same man for the last six years. I met Gavin during the onset of Pat's illness. He knows my brother well and has no fears about our children having a genetic proclivity toward schizophrenia. The odds are on our side.

Environmental factors associated with schizophrenia aren't well understood. Everything from being born in the winter to prenatal depression in the mother has been correlated with development of schizophrenia, but nothing comes close to the predictive power of a family history of the disease. Many illnesses have these risk factors, but by and large, small things aren't enough to account for all cases. For instance, multiple sclerosis is known to occur more frequently the further you get from the equator. This doesn't mean that someone who has lived in Mexico all his or her life can't develop multiple sclerosis. The data, in the end, tell us a great deal and yet not enough.

Although I don't believe that Pat and I grew up in a bad environment, I have often thought about what I can do differently as a parent. The happiness and contentment of a child often correlates with how happy and content his or her parents are. I believe that if I make an effort to be flexible, open to new things, and true to myself, I will be content. I consider my depression to be in remission, and going to therapy has given me some wonderful coping tools if I ever feel myself getting down again. I'm also open to reading more books and getting professional help in the event that I feel like I can't get through the sadness on my own.

Much of my extended family was fraught with noxious interactions. At the same time, I wouldn't want to isolate my children from that. There are all kinds of people in the world. Learning to deal with them is part of life. I think back on a lot of interactions with my relatives and wish that I had handled them differently. Every time a relative's insecurities flared up and they acted rude, angry, unappreciative, or critical, it touched on all my insecurities. I often acted rude and ugly right back at them.

Dealing with my family now, I'm much more secure. I know who I am, and I don't worry about criticism. I try to see my relatives for who they are. My aunts, uncles, cousins, and grandparents didn't have easy lives. None of them had life handed to them on a silver platter. Yes, maybe they behave in ways that put me off, but they will always be my family. Love, especially Grandpa Howard's love, often feels conditional in my family. But I don't want to disown them. That's not who I am. I can't let the way they act change the good person I am. In order to be true to myself, I have to give what I can without thinking about what I can take. Maybe it isn't fair, but life isn't fair.

Since the onset of Pat's illness, I have noticed that he is also much more accepting of our family and all their quirks. He's not critical or dismissive. One incident doesn't speak for a person. He deals with people in the moment. Just because he was annoyed the last time you stopped by doesn't mean he doesn't want to sit and talk with you today. Patience and forgiveness like that are contagious. If you don't hold anything against someone, you'll find that they do the same.

I have thought long and hard about how I will teach my children about schizophrenia. I know that, come what may, they will realize at a young age that Pat is different from other people. If we don't live close to each other, it might take them a little longer. I don't want them to be afraid of him. I will have to bridge the communication gap so that they can get to know him. It's important to me that they understand that he once was a very different man. It had been such a mystery to me that illness could strike in adulthood without any glaring signs. I suppose I thought that people who developed schizophrenia had always been a little strange, a little off. But these things can come from nowhere. Things break. I hope to show my children that we can always pick up the pieces.

I can't control what happens. All I can do is be there for my kids when they need my support. They won't be ignorant of schizophrenia, but they'll know there is no reason to believe that they will have it. I had a great grandmother with Alzheimer's disease. She died when I was six years old. My parents explained to me what the illness was in terms I could understand. Even when we talked about it, when I was older, they never made me feel as though it would happen to me. It's always important to have a "family tree" of illness, but it's not meant to make you feel like you're staring down the barrel of a gun. You can't live your life in fear.

After a while, you get a sense of humor about schizophrenia. One afternoon, helping my mom clean out a junk drawer, I found an old tape recorder. I held it up to her, my eyebrows raised.

"Don't show Pat that!" she squealed.

"I knew it! You've been recording him this whole time!" I shook my head. We laughed and continued cleaning. It might seem inappropriate, but if you can get to a point where you can laugh at something that once scared you so badly it stopped your heart, it is a triumph. That sense of humor has given me new eyes to view the world. Many things don't seem as serious as they once did. We can get through anything, just like we've gotten through everything else.

Being from a family that now has a history of schizophrenia both defines us and says nothing about us at all. Each of us has changed since the diagnosis. But we aren't just a family that schizophrenia *happened* to. We aren't victimized or passively afflicted. We're not obsessively watching for a relapse to happen, but we aren't going to lie down without a fight either. When it comes to facing the future, we are brave because we have to be.

20

Relapse and Healthy Expectations

With the exception of some overarching criteria, the expression of schizophrenia is unique to each person who has it. Pat may not be like any schizophrenic you've ever met. It stands to reason that recovery could look different from case to case too.

Having healthy expectations about Pat's prognosis is something doctors have stressed to us since the beginning. There is no magic pill or special treatment that will suddenly revert a patient back to the way they were before. Once I stopped myself from imagining how things could have been, I started to realize that many of my expectations about Pat's life were superimposed by me. Pat had never had any solid plans for his future. He thought about doing a lot of different things. He had mentioned getting married, and I believe he wanted to have children. But he never dated anyone for very long. He never mentioned that he intended to propose to any of them. He knew his potential, but he didn't have any steadfast prospects for what his future would look like. Now if I jumped in a time machine and asked him at age eighteen if he wanted this life for himself, I don't think he would say yes.

There seems to be a certain amount of disappointment in him that he hasn't done many of the things that his peers have. I think that keeps him from getting in touch with a lot of his old friends. In their early thirties now, many of them went to graduate school, have started careers, and moved away to other cities. Some even have wives and children now. I don't think he wants to explain why he doesn't have those things too. He doesn't realize that he really wouldn't have to explain. I've spoken to many of his friends, and all of them understand the circumstances. What's most difficult is explaining to them why he hasn't returned their calls or e-mails. They feel like Pat doesn't trust them or doesn't like them anymore. I tell them that they can't take it personally. They have a lot of catching up to do, and perhaps he doesn't feel like a long talk the moment they call. Maybe he feels like too much time has passed and maybe they don't want to talk anymore.

In the beginning I had to break the news to many of his friends. Some of them suspected that something was wrong; many had gotten strange phone calls from him while he was delusional. They often ask me how he is, and I tell them without telling them too much. I won't share his life with them in his place. It's not my job to do that. These are his friendships to participate in, not mine.

My expectations for Pat are as flexible as my expectations for other people who are affected by his illness. I can't control the coping mechanisms that other people adopt when they learn about his illness. Some people feel estranged. I can't be sure what he talked to them about when he was delusional, but I can't make apologies for it either. He has had friends who were convinced that Pat was just acting out or using drugs. Denial is probably the easiest way to cope with the diagnosis. All of us want a more tangible reason why he changed so much. We try to reason our way through it, but it just won't budge.

Most of Pat's friends are old friends, people he has known since he was in his formative years. He went to elementary school with them. Because he has not seen them in a long time, since even before his onset, there is the possibility that by now they have grown too far apart. They may not have much in common anymore. It's not just that they have different circumstances, but they have different interests. Pat was always a big fan of music, books, and movies. His tastes have evolved a great deal ever since he started college. One of his favorite things to do is send me an e-mail full of new movies and music to listen to. I reply and send him a list of my own. At times, if we didn't have these exchanges, I don't know what we'd have to talk about.

Our parents probably had more dreams for Pat than I did. It was particularly hard for Dad to accept that Pat has not returned to work and might never take over the family business. It was a source of security he built up for so many years. There was no reason to imagine it wouldn't one day be his son's.

When his friends got married, it wounded Mom. I remember telling her about the wedding of Pat's best friend which I attended in Pennsylvania.

"I hope they all remember their friend. I hope they think about what kind of life he's been left with, after they left him behind," she said.

"You know that isn't fair." I understood her resentment. I used to feel guilty for going on with my own life, as well, as if staying behind would have changed things.

"Well, it seems like they've all forgotten about him."

"What could they do? They couldn't stop him from having schizophrenia."

There was a long silence. "You're right," she sighed. "They have a right to go on with their lives. I'm happy for them."

"They miss him, Mom. I promise you. I know they'd give anything for Pat to be at the wedding, too. I'm sure this isn't how they imagined it."

She sniffled. "He would have made a handsome groomsman."

"I'm sure he would have."

We cannot restore Pat's old friendships for him, no more than I can go back to school or attend his therapy for him. Spurring him on can be difficult, but in the end the responsibility to take action can only be his.

In the end, Pat could have chosen a lot of different paths than the ones we imagined for him. The situation could be worse. He could be in jail, addicted to drugs, or homeless. We could have no relationship with him. We could simply not know where he is or if he's safe. I'll take our circumstances any day over those. If he never developed schizophrenia, maybe he could be a senator, a professor, a husband, or a father. But it's more important to me that he is happy, no matter what he does with his life.

I could let stories I hear in group at NAMI get me down. Incarceration seems to rear its ugly head so often. I've read books by other siblings of schizophrenics, and they often lose touch with their brother or sister entirely. One didn't even know what became of her brother. I don't want to imagine these eventualities for Pat, and I try to keep my expectations for him separate and hopeful.

I've seen every movie I can find on schizophrenia, whether fiction or documentary. Happy endings that come right after the diagnosis seem far-fetched.

"That's just how schizophrenia is for that guy," I think. Delusions and hallucinations were always "solved" by the patient or their doctors, and far too easily I might add. Then it's as if everything will be fine from then on. I realize there's only so much of the story that can be told in 120 minutes, but the Hollywood habit of resolving everything before the credits doesn't serve here. Still, Pat has surprised me so often that I now see the possibility of a happy ending for him too. Our resolutions are small, but they mean everything.

Acceptance of the way things are is something that can come and go. One day I don't mind when I call Pat and he never calls me back. The next time it might hurt my feelings. One day Mom accepts the fact that Pat may never have a family of his own, but later it might make her sad. Dad hires some young men at the office who remind him of Pat when he was just out of college, and then it's harder for him to accept the fact that he's not working with him anymore. I don't see these as setbacks, but rather just as our memories holding on to the way things used to be. And I don't want to forget the old Pat.

Recovery in a clinical sense would mean positive symptoms in remission, management of negative symptoms, regaining the ability to live independently, probably also going back to work, and participating in new or reengaging in old relationships. But that doesn't seem like simple recovery; that seems like recovering *everything*. That seems too absolute, too black and white a definition of recovery. It would be great, but I don't have to experience quite all of that to consider Pat to be in recovery.

I feel that recovery in Pat's case would mean a long period of consistently taking his medication, seeing his psychiatrist, and being open to trying new things, whether that means leaving the house for a short excursion, using the telephone, sending birthday cards, or seeing a new dentist. When he has breakthrough symptoms like delusions of persecution while medicated, I don't think of it as a setback into active psychosis. They're just breaking through. They appear to die down on their own a couple of months later, without any outside intervention other than simply talking to Pat and actively listening to his concerns.

I have noticed how breakthrough symptoms initially made Dr. Russell question everything. He asked a lot of questions to confirm that Pat was still on his medication. He would worry that the medication wasn't working and talk about changing to something else. Then the positive symptoms went away. Now I think he's getting used to the fact that this is just a part of Pat's particular case. His schizophrenia is as unique as he is. This is why I believe his recovery should be unique.

Recovering from schizophrenia shouldn't mean having his life together, getting a job, getting an apartment, and having a girlfriend. Many healthy people don't have their lives that together. I don't have my heart set on the idea that he will one day identify with his diagnosis or start reading up on it. He participates in activities that are meaningful to him. He appears to be happy, to feel safe and secure. He reaches out to us when he needs help with something. I am satisfied with that. As he moves forward and maybe wants more for his life, I can help him move in that direction too. Keeping myself abreast of new medicine and treatments for schizophrenia is a way of arming myself for times ahead. I want Pat to have a great deal of choices in recovery, but all changes are going to happen incrementally. Having a full-scale, mapped-out plan for the future is impossible when you consider relapse and all the forms that can take.

In Pat's case his symptoms flare up seasonally. We've also been careful to moderate his alcohol use because drinking can also contribute to relapse. Big life changes can lead to stress, which also triggers relapse, but his environment is always very calm. There has never been any relapse in his history that followed an instance of a life change or added stress. A young relative passed away since Pat's onset, but there was no relapse at that time or within six months of it. All of his relapses have occurred around the same time of year, November to January, and there has been no pattern among these incidents that tie them together other than the season.

We know to watch for signs of relapse. Any changes in his routine are red flags. Sleep disturbances, changes in appetite, lack of energy, irritability, and shirking responsibilities are all warning signs that positive symptoms are coming. This is probably why it's so hard for caregivers to implement changes in their treatment or day-to-day activities. Change in schizophrenia is often a very bad thing.

Pervasive thinking has always loomed large in Pat's repertoire of episodic behavior. He tends to talk about the same subject over and over again and will not be satisfied with it or allow another person to segue away from it. It's usually rumination on some awkward social situation that he can't seem to cope with after the fact. During the onset of his illness, he would often talk about the same night out he had with his friends right after Hurricane Katrina. But nothing had really happened that night. It was just an ordinary evening. He does a similar thing today during relapse. He harps on a particular event, even if the significance is unclear, and he doesn't want to talk about anything else.

We know where to turn in the event of relapse. We talk to his psychiatrist and talk to other families at NAMI. We know to call 911 in an emergency and ask for police assistance. More than anything, though, we know our roles. We don't overreact or let ourselves become insurmountably stressed. Stress doesn't serve anything other than to exacerbate Pat's paranoia. We take our time with him rather than acting right away.

Often his delusions change shape. They're always persecutory, but they can be very different from the last time. Partnering with him, we listen to his concerns without judgment. It's important to see from his perspective. Because he is firmly convinced that his suspicions are well founded and the persecution is real, we feel his fear and vulnerability. While the delusion isn't real, his feelings are completely genuine. Remembering that makes all the difference.

Before we turn to others for help, we talk to him about it and get a sense for how open he is to sharing his concerns with his psychiatrist. With a kind of "help us help you" approach, we can usually get him to agree to talk with Dr. Russell, but that can take weeks. Without patience and perseverance, we'd never get anywhere.

The first time I found out that Pat had relapsed was after he stopped taking his medication in 2008. I could barely talk to my mom on the phone. I just wanted to cry. I was scared that he'd never accept our help and felt helpless because I was over a thousand miles away from him. I felt disheartened to tell people about the relapse after things had gone so well for a year after the diagnosis. Not everyone realized that things would be different after the relapse, that he wouldn't be able to work or live alone and may never do those things again.

I felt like we were back at square one. But the fact is that we can never go back that far. We've learned too much about Pat and his illness to ever be as naive as we once were. Having been through so much as a family, including the worst hurricane disaster in history, we have tough skin and have bounced back from everything that has come our way. To put it frankly, schizophrenia has no idea who it's dealing with.

The only way to face schizophrenia is to live in the moment instead of harping on what could have been. If things are going well at this point, then I say that things are looking up. It's a far cry from the worst days he's had. It is also important to remember that there are just as many good possibilities for the future as there are bad ones. Recovery is a pastiche of working together, addressing problems one at a time, and trying to find something to be happy about.

In the future, I hope that Pat is capable of living completely independently. I hope he runs his own errands and keeps his appointments. But, as I said before, I don't get too wrapped up in what the future may look like. It's not as if I could have imagined that things would be the way they are now ten years ago.

It worries me that he is dependent upon our father and uncle for his groceries, medication refills, and social activity, because they won't always be around. He says that won't be until years and years from now. "By then I bet I can get anything delivered to my door, even cigarettes."

What I don't ask is, but will they deliver friends?

I don't live nearby, and I have no idea if I will ever move back. Working as a writer in New York is easy, but there are far fewer writing jobs in New Orleans. I have been dating Gavin for nearly seven years, and we talk about starting a family one day. If I put down roots and raise a family outside of New Orleans, I would never be at Pat's disposal.

What if he needs me in the future? Well, I can't imagine he would like me very much as a caregiver. I've never been able to coddle him like our parents do. I certainly wouldn't run his errands unless he came with me. I don't want to do things for him that he is capable of doing himself; I don't want him to be dependent on me for his every need. At this point, I don't think we could live together again. Pat is very untidy.

Financially, I am very happy Dad found the means to provide for Pat. Otherwise I would worry about the burden it would present later on. The trust also requires that spending be regulated by an attorney so that he can't somehow spend or lose it all of a sudden. In providing for myself and my family, I don't know that I could take on Pat, too.

Because he does not leave the house, I worry that if I ever get married Pat will not attend the ceremony. I used to say that I should get married in New Orleans because then he'd be more likely to come, but I fear that's just setting myself up for disappointment. If I plan a New Orleans wedding and he doesn't come, I'll be resentful.

Even worse than missing a wedding, it tears me up thinking that I could have my first child without him coming to meet the baby. I know I would have to wait until I could bring the baby to meet him. It's unfair and sometimes I wish he would make more effort, but I don't know how realistic that expectation is if he's unresponsive to medication.

I don't know what form the future will take for me and my brother, but I know I will work to make it a happy one. I try to be a better person, a smarter person every day. I do what I can to find happiness in the little things. Making that a habit can only bring good things for me and everyone around me, and I hope it rubs off on Pat.

21

Keeping the Friendship Alive

In order to maintain my friendship with Pat, I've had to adapt a great deal. Many of the signs I would read when interacting with another person have to be discounted. He probably won't light up when someone walks into the room, no matter who they are. He may not smile warmly, shake hands, or embrace me. His face is not very expressive. Even when he laughs it's always a quiet chuckle. His body language and demeanor often betray the way he really feels. He can be interested in the conversation without making an enthusiastic face or asking very many questions. It doesn't mean he doesn't want to know.

He doesn't contribute much to conversations, but he's a fairly active listener. Asking him questions usually cuts the conversation short. His answers are usually vague. There is not a great deal of fluidity in his speech, as part of the negative symptom called alogia. If Pat is rambling, then something is definitely wrong. I have to do most of the talking. I don't mind carrying the social load, if he feels like he is getting something out of all my babbling. It's worth it for the occasions when he does volunteer information and seems to enjoy talking about himself and his hobbies.

He might break off from a conversation and go outside to have a quick smoke or take care of his cat. His intention is to return to talking later, but by then a person might be getting ready to leave. This wouldn't necessarily disappoint him. He'd just say, "We'll talk next time."

If someone else did this to me, I'd think they didn't like me very much. I have to check my hang-ups at the door. Taking it personally when he seems disinterested or unengaged is silly. If I feel like he wants to be left alone, I have to just come out and ask him. His answer is usually no.

Because his demeanor is fairly static, there is no reason to be so sensitive to it. It can be difficult to resist getting my feelings hurt sometimes, but it's just my own insecurities bleeding through. I have to put my need for approval on the shelf and accept the fact that I truly don't know what he's thinking. Learning to accept this has been liberating. I'm a better communicator when I'm not spending all my time attending to every little movement of his face. I am more myself now when I speak to him than I could have been before.

Everyone has quirks. In human relations, we all bring something different to the table, whether you're a neat freak, a prude, or an intellectual. Some people prefer not to talk about certain things. Some subjects fray nerves or pick at the chip on your shoulder. Some people don't open up easily and others have to draw them out carefully. Other people are boisterous or excited to share. We can't get along with everyone. In fact most people don't relish being in socially awkward situations. Being around a schizophrenic can feel like that all the time. But the expectations for dealing with others have to be changed, not lowered, when you speak to a schizophrenic. You must be patient, reach out to them, and not overreact if you're rebuffed. You have to get comfortable with them giving vague or unusual answers to questions. This might even mean ignoring their hygiene or strange movements.

If Pat says something that sounds judgmental or off-putting, it's usually a misread and not intended that way. There are times in the past when he was trying to show interest in things, but it sounded like he was being pushy or sarcastic. I brought my dog with me once on a visit, and Pat spent the whole time giving him pieces of roasted chicken from the fridge. I warned him to stop because the dog's stomach was sensitive. Eventually the dog threw it all up, and I was obviously annoyed.

To this day whenever I visit, he asks, "Where's the dog?" Initially I thought he was being sarcastic or mean, but when I asked him, I realized he barely remembers the time he fed my dog scraps until he puked. He was asking out of genuine interest in who was watching my dog while I was visiting.

Mom and Dad have also had conversations with Pat where they thought he was being caustic and disrespectful. When his responses sound curt and he seems like he has better things to do than talk, it's easy to misconstrue this for a slight.

We learned over time that the things we think we hear or see in Pat are often just our own insecurities filling in the blanks. No one wants to think that in communicating with someone they are making them bored or annoyed. It's just not in our nature to enjoy feeling bothersome to another person. We try to take cues from others and let that guide our interactions, but Pat just doesn't put out much in the way of cues.

As an introvert, I don't measure the scope of his recovery by how much Pat seems to want to socialize. I can sympathize with the fact that talking to people can be exhausting. Trying to find something to say, to actively listen and respond, is not something that ever came easy for me. I respect my brother's wishes to be left alone sometimes and don't consider it to be a negative quality. Recovery shouldn't mean that all his quirks go away. It doesn't mean being agreeable or accommodating in social situations. He has been a straight shooter his whole life. He never wasted words, told white lies, or lavished someone with compliments. On the other hand, he wasn't overly critical or assumptive. He just treated others the way he wanted to be treated in return.

When we were young Pat was very extroverted. He was friends with everyone in his grade and a few that were older than him, too. Most people would have described him as funny. Sometimes he could be a little cocky, but it often came off as charming.

Seeming interested in what someone is saying even when you aren't is a skill many people have to use every day. Pat just never got the hang of it, even before the onset. I joke with him about it sometimes, but he just smiles and shrugs. It never made much sense to him that people exchange niceties; to him it's simply a waste of time. He doesn't get any joy from having a short how-do-you-do with someone. If it's someone he doesn't know very well, it's even more superfluous. "We don't know each other. Why should I pretend to care about him?" he would say.

He still doesn't like to use the phone, and when I text him, I often don't hear back. I just have to know that he will see my messages at some point. I respond to his messages quickly and don't mind if he never responds to mine. I still send him texts about movies to watch and music to buy. In 2012, we watched the presidential debates and texted each other back and forth. I'm comfortable with the fact that he often only wants to talk about things that interest him and doesn't ask a lot about things that only interest me. I guess I am lucky we still have so much in common.

If I visit him and he doesn't have much to say, I'll go to his room. He always leaves the door open. He sits watching TV, sometimes with his fat cat in his lap. I sit on the bed and watch something with him. We'll talk a little, and he seems to enjoy the company. I think some people don't realize how easy it is. Maybe they think going into his room is invading his space. Instead it's just a place he feels most comfortable.

If he is relapsing, he may stick on a certain subject. It's a sign of pervasive thinking again. I do my best to talk about other things, but I can't push too hard. I don't want him to feel as though he can't talk to me about something. Knowing his thoughts is a key component to seeing how he arrives at a delusion, the culmination of obsessive and paranoid thoughts.

Otherwise, Pat is usually quiet and reserved. I know that one way to get him talking is to annoy him somehow. MTV had brought back a silly, toilet-humor cartoon that we used to watch when we were kids called *Beavis and Butthead*. When I heard the news, I sent a text to both Pat and Dad, who also used to watch the cartoon with us sometimes. I didn't expect to hear back, but a week or so later, I got a series of messages from Pat.

PAT: Why did you tell Dad about the new season of *Beavis and Butthead* and not me? Who is the bigger fan? I own all three volumes of the Mike Judge collection and *Beavis and Butthead Do America*.

ME: I did tell you. Scroll up on your text messages.

PAT: Oh, I see.

ME: Well now I know all I have to do is piss you off to get you to text me three whole sentences. The secret is out!

PAT: You might be right. . . . I still love you though.

ME: I love you too!

That put a huge smile on my face. I knew then he was back. That was such a Pat reaction through and through. I showed the text to my boyfriend and he said, "Wow, he's just like you when he's annoyed."

It is very painful to think that lurking behind the health is an illness that will not ever be cured. But I know schizophrenia's tricks. I know it's strong and unpredictable, but schizophrenia never met a sister with more strength and resilience. It's taken Pat from us before, but we will never stop fighting to get him back.

He still says things sometimes like he's looking at our family, our lives, for the first time. He used to love getting into political debates with our dad. They could go on and on for hours. I didn't like it. I was afraid it would get too heated.

Recently he said, "Dad really doesn't see eye to eye with me on politics."

Mom and I look at him quizzically. "You mean, like always?" I asked.

"I guess so." He just shrugged like he didn't have a personal history with Dad, a frame of reference. It can be sad, when he seems to be out of practice in dealing with people he has known his whole life, but it's also comforting that he's engaged in his family relationships again.

He lost some time, so to speak, to active psychosis. When he is delusional he doesn't think much about things that happen on the news or even events going on in his own life. He focuses squarely on his delusions and what he can do about them. He's too anxious and amped up to pay attention to anything else. It's not unlike intense anxiety that any person feels when something goes wrong in life. If you lost your job and had a family to support, thinking about what to do to rectify that can consume you. Pat is similarly consumed by his delusions of persecution.

Because of these periods, I've had to do some filling in for him of the last few years. These longer messages I usually e-mail to him. I told him about the circumstances of our parents' divorce. While he knew they had been unhappy and that they were now divorced, he didn't know how that unfolded. He missed it even though it was happening right before his eyes.

I told him about the classes I took. Most of the time I was in graduate school, Pat was unresponsive to the medications he was prescribed. Much of 2008 is a blur for him. I told him about what it was like to live in Bed-Stuy, Brooklyn, when the first black president of the United States was elected. There were parties in the street nearly all night long.

In the last few years I've written some freelance articles online for news outlets and blogs. I even had my novel thesis published in 2011. While Pat hasn't read any of this recent work, he likes when I tell him about it. He doesn't really read any fiction, but if I'm in the middle of a good book, he likes when I tell him about the story. He tells me what the book reminds him of and might recommend some others to me.

It took me a long time to let go of my fears that I might tell Pat something that would fuel his anxiety or make him paranoid. I can't help the fact that he can have delusions and that he might use information I have discussed with him as evidence that they are real. There is no way to know what he will or will not take away from our conversations. I can't let that stand in the way of keeping our relationship active and healthy.

After I saw Darren Aronofsky's film *Black Swan*, I didn't know what to do. I thought it was one of the most genuine attempts to give an audience a front-row seat to the confusion and terror in the mind of a person descending into schizophrenia. I was enthralled by it, and knowing how much Pat loves psychological thrillers, I thought he would appreciate it too. So many questions filled my head: But what if he identifies with it and finds it embarrassing? What if he doesn't identify with it and decides he doesn't want to take medication anymore? What if he thinks I'm trying to communicate something to him by suggesting it to him, like a code? I gave up. The possibilities were endless. He saw the film and thought it was great. That's all there was to it.

There's something about being enveloped in anxiety, fears of being persecuted, for so many years and having little distraction or even energy for anything else that seems to unravel many of the memories Pat once had. Memory deficits are a feature of his illness. People with schizophrenia may process information differently from the rest of us, making it difficult to make and retrieve long-term memories. Helping Pat to remember things or fill in the blanks has led to something I refer to as identity talk. He hasn't talked much about his personal history in many years. Sometimes, when he's having a good day, I find him volunteering information when talking to people, showing not only that he is more introspective now, but also that he feels he can trust us.

It may not seem fair that our interactions don't have a balance of give and take, but I don't mind. That's not what motivates me to talk with him in the first place. Much of the encouragement and advice that I once needed from my big brother is already with me, every day. I can parse out what he would think or what he would say about things. I don't need him to "open up" that way. Instead, I enjoy hearing him say as much or as little as he wants about whatever. Sometimes keeping the friendship alive is making the effort and helping him meet his needs. He may not talk to me about anything particularly heavy, but I'm not afraid to. And I make sure he knows I love him and I'm not going anywhere.

Resources

I spent a great deal of time trying to find information and real-life stories on schizophrenia. Things I've listed below are those that resonated with me the most. I am more knowledgeable because of them and also inspired by them.

Personally, I'm not sure how anyone managed to find resources on schizophrenia before the Internet. I left so many unanswered phone calls with psychologists and psychiatrists, it's a wonder we ever got Pat the help he needed. Today answers might be a keystroke away.

I found that getting through schizophrenia in one piece requires finding support for yourself. It will make you a much better support for your loved one. Don't bury your emotions. Find a way to let them out. I have found that writing about Pat's schizophrenia on an online blog has helped me a great deal to organize my thoughts and emotions over the last six years. Finding a way to communicate and sort out my feelings has been a great help in the coping process.

ORGANIZATIONS AND WEBSITES

The LEAP Institute
P.O. Box 29
Peconic, NY 11958
Information: (800) 801-LEAP (5327)
www.leapinstitute.org

National Alliance on Mental Illness (NAMI)
3803 N. Fairfax Dr., Suite 100
Arlington, VA 22203-1701
Main: (703) 524-7600
Member Services: (888) 999-6264
Help Line: (800) 950-6264

Brain and Behavior Research Foundation
60 Cutter Mill Road, Suite 404
Great Neck, NY 11021-3131
Help Line: (800) 829-8289
bbrfoundation.org

The National Institute of Mental Health (NIMH)
Science Writing, Press, and Dissemination Branch
6001 Executive Blvd., Room 6200, MSC 9663
Bethesda, MD 20892-9663
(866) 615-6464
www.nimh.nih.gov

American Psychiatric Association (APA)
1000 Wilson Blvd., Suite 1825
Arlington, VA 22209-3901
(888) 35-PSYCH (77924)
www.psych.org

Film is one of my favorite mediums. Documentaries on schizophrenia offer a one-of-a-kind glimpse into the lives of those who struggle and cope with it every day.

FAVORITE DOCUMENTARY FILMS

Out of the Shadow. Dir. Susan Smiley (Vine Street Pictures, 2004). This documentary follows the life of the director's mother, Millie Smiley, who has struggled with schizophrenia since adolescence. It is a great resource on schizophrenia, aging, and family relationships.

People Say I'm Crazy. Dir. John Cadigan and Katie Cadigan (HBO/Cinemax Documentary Films, 2003). A brave documentary from a man diagnosed with schizophrenia at age twenty-one. With the help of his sister Katie, John Cadigan tells us the story of his illness, recovery, and strong family support. Illuminating, this story made me look at aspects of psychosis I never imagined before.

Wesley Willis: The Daddy of Rock 'n' Roll. Dir. Daniel Bitton (Music Video Distributors, 2003). Filmed in 2000, this documentary follows the day-to-day struggles of influential African American musician Wesley Willis due to schizophrenia and a weight disorder. Willis heard voices and spent much of his life homeless on the streets of Chicago playing music and selling his drawings. Willis's endless creativity and soulfulness are inspirational.

Some books on schizophrenia can center on treatment and use technical jargon that can be hard to digest. Below are the books I found to be the most readable, useful, and relatable.

HELPFUL BOOKS TO START WITH

Amador, Xavier. *I'm Not Sick, I Don't Need Help!* (Peconic, NY: Vida Press, 2012). Dr. Xavier Amador, a clinical psychologist and Columbia University professor, writes about how to help people with mental illness accept treatment. He developed the LEAP method from his own experience with his brother's schizophrenia and thirty years of clinical experience. This is one of the only books I've read that offers simple tools for talking persuasively with someone who refuses treatment.

Torrey, E. Fuller. *Surviving Schizophrenia: A Manual for Families, Consumers, and Providers* (New York: HarperCollins, 2001). Dr. Torrey's manual is the primary resource for my family. Full of information on the development of schizophrenia, possible outcomes, and treatment, this is a book I return to time and again.

BOOKS BY PEOPLE WITH SCHIZOPHRENIA OR THEIR FAMILY MEMBERS

Bennett, Amanda, and Lori Schiller. *The Quiet Room: A Journey Out of the Torment of Madness* (New York: Warner Books, 1994). This book is a personal account of author Lori Schiller who in her early twenties found herself wandering New York City tormented by voices in her head.

Greenburg, Hannah (originally under the pen name Hannah Green). *I Never Promised You a Rose Garden* (New York: Holt, 1964). This semiautobiographical novel was one of the first of its kind. Its main character is a teenage girl diagnosed with schizophrenia, institutionalized and fighting to regain her sanity.

Kaye, Randye. *Ben behind His Voices: One Family's Journey from the Chaos of Schizophrenia to Hope* (Lanham, MD: Rowman & Littlefield, 2011). Author Randye Kaye writes about her son Ben's schizophrenia and her family's struggle to cope.

Neugeboren, Jay. *Imagining Robert: My Brother, Madness, and Survival, a Memoir* (New Brunswick, NJ: Rutgers University Press, 1997). Neugeboren has written a number of novels, and his prose is a real delight to read. He has always been very close with his brother Robert, who suffered a mental breakdown when he was eighteen years old.

Simon, Clea. *Madhouse: Growing Up in the Shadow of Mentally Ill Siblings* (New York: Penguin, 1998). Simon gives an autobiographical account of growing up in a family with two older siblings, her brother and her sister, both diagnosed with schizophrenia.

If you find that learning some history on schizophrenia and mental health services lends a great deal of perspective, the following might interest you.

FURTHER READING

Beam, Alex. *Gracefully Insane: Life and Death Inside America's Premier Mental Hospital* (New York: PublicAffairs, 2001). Beam takes us inside the once-prestigious McLean Hospital where Ray Charles, Sylvia Plath, and John Nash were patients. The history of this hospital traces both the failures and great triumphs of psychiatric services in the United States.

Penney, Darby, and Peter Stastny. *The Lives They Left Behind: Suitcases from a State Hospital Attic* (New York: Bellevue Literary Press, 2008). Over four hundred suitcases were found at the Willard Psychiatric Center after it was closed in the early 1990s. The authors use the articles inside to piece together the lives these patients led before they were institutionalized.

Torrey, E. Fuller. *The Insanity Offense: How America's Failure to Treat the Seriously Mentally Ill Endangers Its Citizens* (New York: Norton, 2012). Torrey, who wrote *Surviving Schizophrenia*, compiles historical data and the court cases that led to deinstitutionalization and examines how that change affected the vulnerable population of people with schizophrenia and the communities in which they live.

OTHER WEBSITES AND PUBLICATIONS

Schizophrenia Research Forum (www.schizophreniaforum.org). This is a website for mental health consumers, caregivers, and researchers in the area of schizophrenia to share information, news, and expertise.

SZ Magazine (www.mentalwellnesstoday.com). Diagnosed with schizophrenia at age twenty-four, editor Bill McPhee began this magazine in 1994. It includes columns from individuals with schizophrenia as well as research news and tips on coping. The website also includes articles on schizophrenia, bipolar disorder, and depression.

Schizophrenia.com (www.schizophrenia.com) offers a wealth of resources, news, tips on coping, and even forums where parents, siblings, and other caregivers can post and ask for feedback from the rest of the community.

Acknowledgments

Thank you to my big brother for letting me tell his story, for always humoring me, and for all the ways he continues to surprise and inspire us all. Thank you to my parents for always encouraging me to write and for helping me tell our story in these pages. Their support and openness to this project have helped me discover the most significant milestones in our family's journey through schizophrenia.

Words cannot describe the amount of help I have received from the National Alliance on Mental Illness. The level of compassion I found there was unmatched. With NAMI I not only found training on how to help Pat but also how to help myself. I realized that without caring for myself, I was no use to him. I now have strategies for dealing with relapse, negative symptoms, and the way the illness affects Pat's friends and our family.

For helping me realize this book, a special thanks to Suzanne Staszak-Silva, the senior acquisitions editor at Rowman & Littlefield Publishers and all the care their staff has taken to make it wonderful.

Notes

INTRODUCTION

1. "Report: Who's Watching?" New York Civil Liberties Union, http://www.nyclu
.org/publications/report-whos-watching-2006 (accessed June 10, 2012).

CHAPTER 2

1. Richard J. Lewine and Elaine Walker, "Prediction of Adult-Onset Schizophrenia
from Childhood Home Movies of Patients," *American Journal of Psychiatry* 147, no.
8 (1990): 1052.

CHAPTER 5

1. Stacy Shaw Welch, "A Review of the Literature on the Epidemiology of
Parasuicide in the General Population," *Psychiatric Services* 52, no. 3 (2001): 368.

CHAPTER 7

1. E. Fuller Torrey, *Surviving Schizophrenia: A Manual for Families, Consumers,
and Providers* (New York: HarperCollins, 2001), 98.

CHAPTER 11

1. "A Short Introduction to Schizophrenia," Schizophrenia.com, http://www
.schizophrenia.com/family/schizintro.html (accessed January 13, 2013).

2. Leslie Citrome and Jan Volavka, "The Promise of Atypical Antipsychotics: Fewer Side Effects Mean Enhanced Compliance and Improved Functioning," *Postgraduate Medicine* 116, no. 4 (2004): 49.

3. Christoph U. Correll et al., "Cardiometabolic Risk of Second-Generation Antipsychotic Medications during First-Time Use in Children and Adolescents," *Journal of the American Medical Association* 302, no. 16 (October 2009): 1765, doi:10.1001/jama.2009.1549.

4. Jennifer Berg, Gregory Stajich, and Martin Zdanowicz, "Atypical Antipsychotic-Induced Type 2 Diabetes," *Pharmacy Times*, March 14, 2012, http://www.pharmacytimes.com/publications/issue/2012/March2012/Olanzapine-and-clozapine-Atypical-Antipsychotic-Induced-Type-2-Diabetes-.

5. K. Saari et al., "Hyperlipidemia in Persons Using Antipsychotic Medication: A General Population-Based Birth Cohort Study," *Journal of Clinical Psychiatry* 65, no. 4 (2004): 547.

6. "Schizophrenia Facts and Statistics," Schizophrenia.com, http://www.schizophrenia.com/szfacts.htm (accessed February 19, 2013).

7. "Schizophrenia," National Institute of Mental Health, last modified 2009, http://www.nimh.nih.gov/health/publications/schizophrenia/index.shtml.

8. E. Fuller Torrey, *Surviving Schizophrenia: A Manual for Families, Consumers, and Providers* (New York: HarperCollins, 2001), 367.

9. Dennis K. Kinney et al., "Relation of Schizophrenia Prevalence to Latitude, Climate, Fish Consumption, Infant Mortality, and Skin Color: A Role for Prenatal Vitamin D Deficiency and Infections?" *Schizophrenia Bulletin* 35, no. 3 (2009): 582.

10. Filippo Varese et al., "Childhood Adversities Increase the Risk of Psychosis: A Meta-analysis of Patient-Control, Prospective- and Cross-Sectional Cohort Studies," *Schizophrenia Bulletin* 38, no. 4 (2012): 661.

11. Filip Smit, Linda Bolier, and Pim Cuijpers, "Cannabis Use and the Risk of Later Schizophrenia: A Review," *Addiction* 99, no. 4 (2004): 429–30.

CHAPTER 12

1. J. Bustillo et al., "The Psychosocial Treatment of Schizophrenia: An Update," *American Journal of Psychiatry* 158, no. 2 (2001): 163.

2. Thomas A. Richards, "What Is Comprehensive Cognitive Behavioral Therapy?" Social Anxiety Institute website, http://www.socialanxietyinstitute.org/ccbtherapy.html (accessed December 11, 2012).

3. M. I. Gutierrez-Lopez et al., "Cognitive Behavioral Therapy for Chronic Psychosis," *Actas Espanolas de Psiquiatria* 37, no. 2 (2009): 106.

CHAPTER 17

1. "Refractory Schizophrenia," Schizophrenia.com, http://www.schizophrenic.com/articles/schizophrenia/refractory-schizophrenia (accessed February 27, 2003).

CHAPTER 18

1. D. Folsom and D. V. Jeste, "Schizophrenia in Homeless Persons: A Systematic Review of the Literature," *Acta Psychiatrica Scandinavica* 105, no. 6 (June 2002): 405.

2. Alan R. Felthous, "The Involuntary Medication of Jared Loughner and Pretrial Jail Detainees in Nonmedical Correctional Facilities," *Journal of the American Academy of Psychiatry and the Law* 40 (2012): 98.

3. E. Fuller Torrey, *The Insanity Offense: How America's Failure to Treat the Seriously Mentally Ill Endangers Its Citizens* (New York: Norton, 2012), 53.

4. M. Pompili et al., "Suicide Risk in Schizophrenia: Learning from the Past to Change the Future," *Annals of General Psychiatry* 6, no. 10 (March 16, 2007), doi:10.1186/1744-859X-6-10.

CHAPTER 19

1. E. Fuller Torrey, *Surviving Schizophrenia: A Manual for Families, Consumers, and Providers* (New York: HarperCollins, 2001), 144.

Bibliography

American Psychiatric Association. *Diagnostic and Statistical Manual of Mental Disorders*. 4th ed. rev. (DSM-IV-TR). Washington, DC: American Psychiatric Association, 2000. doi:10.1176/appi.books.9780890423349.

Berg, Jennifer, Gregory Stajich, and Martin Zdanowicz. "Atypical Antipsychotic-Induced Type 2 Diabetes." *Pharmacy Times*, March 14, 2012. http://www.pharmacytimes.com/publications/issue/2012/March2012/Olanzapine-and-clozapine-Atypical-Antipsychotic-Induced-Type-2-Diabetes-.

Bustillo, J., J. Lauriello, W. Horan, and S. Keith. "The Psychosocial Treatment of Schizophrenia: An Update." *American Journal of Psychiatry* 158, no. 2 (2001): 163–75.

Citrome, Leslie, and Jan Volavka. "The Promise of Atypical Antipsychotics: Fewer Side Effects Mean Enhanced Compliance and Improved Functioning." *Postgraduate Medicine* 116, no. 4 (2004): 49–51, 55–59, 63.

Correll, Christoph U., Peter Manu, Vladimir Olshanskiy, Barbara Napolitano, John M. Kane, and Anil K. Malhotra. "Cardiometabolic Risk of Second-Generation Antipsychotic Medications during First-Time Use in Children and Adolescents." *Journal of the American Medical Association* 302, no. 16 (October 2009): 1765–73. doi:10.1001/jama.2009.1549.

Felthous, Alan R. "The Involuntary Medication of Jared Loughner and Pretrial Jail Detainees in Nonmedical Correctional Facilities." *Journal of the American Academy of Psychiatry and the Law* 40 (2012): 98–112.

Folsom, D., and D. V. Jeste. "Schizophrenia in Homeless Persons: A Systematic Review of the Literature." *Acta Psychiatrica Scandinavica* 105, no. 6 (June 2002): 404–13.

Gutierrez-Lopez, M. I., M. Sanchez Munoz, A. Trujilo Borrego, and L. Sanchez Bonome. "Cognitive Behavioral Therapy for Chronic Psychosis." *Actas Espanolas de Psiquiatria* 37, no. 2 (2009): 106–14.

Kinney, Dennis K., Pamela Teixeira, Diane Hsu, Siena C. Napoleon, David J. Crowley, Andrew Miller, William Hyman, and Emerald Huang. "Relation of Schizophrenia Prevalence to Latitude, Climate, Fish Consumption, Infant Mortality, and Skin Color: A Role for Prenatal Vitamin D Deficiency and Infections?" *Schizophrenia Bulletin* 35, no. 3 (2009): 582–95.

Lewine, Richard J., and Elaine Walker. "Prediction of Adult-Onset Schizophrenia from Childhood Home Movies of Patients." *American Journal of Psychiatry* 147, no. 8 (1990): 1052–56.

National Institute of Mental Health. "Schizophrenia." Last modified 2009. http://www.nimh.nih.gov/health/publications/schizophrenia/index.shtml.

New York Civil Liberties Union. "Report: Who's Watching?" http://www.nyclu.org/publications/report-whos-watching-2006 (accessed June 10, 2012).

Pompili, M., X. F. Amador, P. Girardi, J. Harkavy-Friedman, M. Harrow, K. Kaplan, et al. "Suicide Risk in Schizophrenia: Learning from the Past to Change the Future." *Annals of General Psychiatry* 6, no. 10 (March 16, 2007). doi:10.1186/1744-859X-6-10.

Richards, Thomas A. "What Is Comprehensive Cognitive Behavioral Therapy?" Social Anxiety Institute website. http://www.socialanxietyinstitute.org/ccbtherapy.html (accessed December 11, 2012).

Saari, K., H. Koponen, J. Laitinen, J. Jokelainen, L. Lauren, M. Isohanni, and S. Lindeman. "Hyperlipidemia in Persons Using Antipsychotic Medication: A General Population-Based Birth Cohort Study." *Journal of Clinical Psychiatry* 65, no. 4 (2004): 547–50.

Schizophrenia.com. "Refractory Schizophrenia." http://www.schizophrenic.com/articles/schizophrenia/refractory-schizophrenia (accessed February 27, 2013).

———. "Schizophrenia Facts and Statistics." http://www.schizophrenia.com/szfacts.htm (accessed February 19, 2013).

———. "A Short Introduction to Schizophrenia." http://www.schizophrenia.com/family/schizintro.html (accessed January 13, 2013).

Smit, Filip, Linda Bolier, and Pim Cuijpers. "Cannabis Use and the Risk of Later Schizophrenia: A Review." *Addiction* 99, no. 4 (2004): 425–30.

Torrey, E. Fuller. *The Insanity Offense: How America's Failure to Treat the Seriously Mentally Ill Endangers Its Citizens.* New York: Norton, 2012.

———. *Surviving Schizophrenia: A Manual for Families, Consumers, and Providers.* New York: HarperCollins, 2001.

Varese, Filippo, Feikje Smeets, Marjan Drukker, Ritsaert Lieverse, Tineke Lataster, Wolfgang Viechtbauer, et al. "Childhood Adversities Increase the Risk of Psychosis: A Meta-analysis of Patient-Control, Prospective- and Cross-Sectional Cohort Studies." *Schizophrenia Bulletin* 38, no. 4 (2012): 661–71.

Welch, Stacy Shaw. "A Review of the Literature on the Epidemiology of Parasuicide in the General Population." *Psychiatric Services* 52, no. 3 (2001): 368–75.

About the Author

Sarah Rae is a writer and an editor. She is the author of *Charity*, a novel about five families during Hurricane Katrina. Her fiction and nonfiction have appeared in literary journals internationally since 2006. A member of the Freelancers Union, she writes and copyedits web content. She is also the editor-in-chief of a literary journal. She blogs about schizophrenia at www.fogofparanoia.com.